THE PT WEBSITE

SECRETS™

SYSTEM

GET THE SECRET FORMULA TO WIN MORE PATIENTS & MAKE MORE PROFIT FROM YOUR PT WEBSITE

Christine Walker

Publisher: Christine Walker, 8850 Monroe Road, Charlotte, NC 28212

While they have made every effort to verify the information here, neither the author nor the publisher assumes any responsibility for errors in, omissions from or a different interpretation of the subject matter. This information may be subject to varying laws and practices in different areas, states, and countries. The reader assumes all responsibility for the use of the information.

The author and publisher shall in no event be held liable to any party for any damages arising directly or indirectly from any use of this material. Every effort that been made to accurately represent this product and its potential and there is no guarantee that you will earn any money using these techniques.

ISBN: 978-1-7908-5635-0

DEDICATION

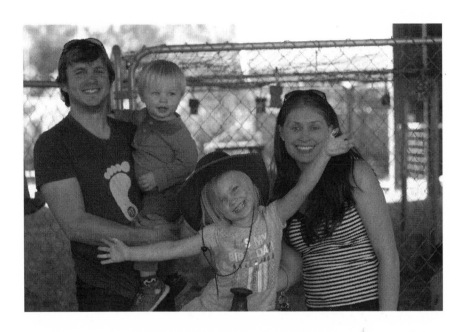

To David, Virginia, & Jackson.
My Family. My Cheerleaders. My Inspiration.
I Love You All So Much.

To My Clients.
Thank you for joining me on this journey,
and for inviting me on yours.

Thank You God.
The greatest author of all.

BEFORE YOU READ THIS BOOK, DO THIS FIRST...

[DOWNLOAD A GIFT FROM CHRISTINE - A $1297 VALUE!]

As a thanks for reading this book, **I want to give you some awesome bonuses** to help you implement what you'll learn in this book into your PT business - **all for FREE!**

To Download, Go To:

www.ptwebsitesecretsbook.com/resources

Here's What You'll Receive:

1. **The 6 PT Website Secrets™ Questions Worksheet**
2. **The 7 Must-Ask Questions To Get Great Patient Testimonials**
3. **Worksheet: The 4 Must-Ask (And Often Forgotten) Questions To Finding Your Ideal Patient Group**
4. **Scorecard For Tracking Your Website's Success**

   <u>AND</u> *(The Most Anticipated Gift)*

5. **The Tips from My Back Pain Report Copyright-Free!** *(A $997 Value by Itself!)*

Get Your Gift Here:

www.ptwebsitesecretsbook.com/resources

AS YOU READ THIS BOOK, YOU'RE GOING TO WANT TO HAVE THESE...

Go To www.ptwebsitesecretsbook.com/resources **now and download your FREE bonus gift worth $1297 so that you can get the MOST out of this book and start changing your business today!**

PRAISE FOR PT WEBSITE SECRETS™

"Christine's success in helping PT Clinic owners build a profitable website has been nothing short of sensational. The impact that Christine will have upon your clinics success extends way beyond just having a more profitable website, and I wholeheartedly recommend you at least speak to her to find out what she can do for you."

Paul Gough – Author, Founder of *Paul Gough Media* & *Paul Gough Physio Rooms*, Hartlepool, UK

"Christine has the best formula when it comes to having a website that actually makes you money and gets you customers!"

Greg Todd – Career & Business Consultant for PTs, Co-Owner *Renewal Rehabilitation*, Tampa, FL

"If you want a website that converts visitors into cash paying patients, then look no further than the website wizard herself, Christine Walker!"

Aaron LeBauer, *LeBauer Physical Therapy*, Greensboro, NC

"If anyone asks us for website help, we send them straight to Christine! Christine makes it really clear why your website isn't working! Christine gave me more actionable website changes in 5 minutes than I could come up with after staring at it for 4 days! Trust me, don't waste time trying to 'figure it out' on your own, just go learn from Christine!"

Alex Engar - *Healthcare Digital Marketing*, *Healthy Funnel* Podcast, Salt Lake City, UT

"Before working with Christine, I was stressed and relying on doctor referrals and weekend events to get new patients. My old website was more or less an online brochure. My new *PT Website Secrets*™ website is an active, integrated, lead-generating machine! It gets us at least 5 new patients each week!"

Paul Jones, *Jones Physical Therapy*, New Orleans, LA

"I've had such a great experience working with Christine and *PT Website Secrets*™. With the changes she made, we get 1-2 new patients from our website each week... that's going to add $40,000 to our bottom line this year. Thank you!"

Kris Winders, *BBN Physical Therapy*, Lexington, KY

"I can't believe it! My old website did nothing for my business. With my new *PT Website Secrets*™ I've gotten 13 leads in 2 months, and 10 have become patients. I now get calls consistently from my perfect patient. This is super exciting for me!"

Chad Cohle, *Cohle Chiro*, Harrisburg, PA

"I spent years with a website that did nothing. Right after launching my new *PT Website Secrets*™ website, I have my first new patient from online!"

Laura McKaig, *Laura McKaig Physical Therapy*, Overland Park, KS

"I highly recommend Christine and *PT Website Secrets*™. Before, I was getting zero calls from my website. Now, I get calls and the people coming in are more prepared to buy than before. It's allowed me to add extra income WITHOUT working harder! Thank you again, Christine!"

John Davidson, Jr., *Calso Physical Therapy*, Greensboro, NC.

"Before implementing the *PT Website Secrets™ System*, I got about at most 3-4 patient inquiries a month from my website... now I get 3-4 A WEEK!"

Cameron Dennis, *Back On Track Physical Therapy & Wellness*, **Wapakoneta, OH**

"Christine Walker (AKA the PT Website Wizard) is the only person to guide you through the creation of your direct response website! She chunks every section down into easy-to-do tasks and allowed a total technophobe to achieve website success!!!!"

Emma Green, Pasadena, CA

"Christine makes the process of transforming your website so smooth. It has really empowered me and enhanced my self-confidence by recognizing the value that I can provide to patients. I cannot thank you enough!"

Tony Farina, *Impact Performance Therapy*, **Columbus, OH**

"I knew I needed to make significant changes to my practice website in order to attract the type of patients I was looking for, but the task of doing so always seemed so daunting! The *"PTWS System* made it easy and intuitive for me to break down the necessary parts, create the content, and ultimately create a direct response website that attracts my ideal customer."

Brooke Kalisiak, *Legacy Physical Therapy*, **St. Louis, MO**

"Working with Christine and her *PT Website Secrets™ System* was a hugely impactful move and one of the best decisions I've made in the early growth stage of my PT business. She walked me through the entire process from start to finish and has shown a genuine interest in the results that it has brought in. She's providing a much-needed service to the world of PT business owners!"

Debbie Cohen, *Fundamental Physical Therapy & Pelvic Wellness*, **San Diego, CA**

"While some may understand the ins and outs of what *should* be on their website, even fewer understand what *must* be included for their website to be a functioning, lead generating asset. Christine did an excellent job not only setting up my website, but also putting together the backend aspects that make a website a valuable marketing asset and not just a homepage."

Marc Luko, *Optimal Performance & Reconditioning*, D.C.

"For the first time I got a new patient from online! I can't believe the results I'm getting from my website!"

Joann Pung, *Manual Physical Therapy &*
***Concierge Services*, Sarasota, FL**

"In my second week of business I just sold my first package at $247 a visit – and the patient came from the website I made with the *PT Website Secrets™ System!*"

Joshua Hall, *Hall Physical Therapy*, Salt Lake City, UT

"The *PT Website Secrets™ Workshop* is one of the best investment I ever made!"

Nuha Hassan, *Ascend Physical Therapy*, Orland Park, IL

"The *PT Website Secrets™ Workshop* course is AMAZING! You've made the process of transforming my website such a breeze. Thank you so much!"

Elena Johnson, Denver, CO

"Before, I was stuck working as a contractor and unable to grow my location efficiently and effectively. Now, I'm 100% on my own, have my own *PT Website Secrets™* website, am making more money, and am now able to spend the time needed to develop the business. I'm excited to finally get my practice where I want it to be!"

Jamie So, *Manual Therapy Effects*, McLean, VA

"Christine's system has totally changed my mindset and future outlook for my business!"

Matt Longfellow, Columbus, OH

"After working with Christine, my website worked for me, so I had to do less work on my end to nurture my leads. This freed my time for higher dollar value tasks."

Jack Wong, *Next Level Physical Therapy*, Houston, TX

"Christine and her team make the process of creating a lead generating website simple and streamlined. Their feedback and guidance throughout the process are invaluable."

Dr Beth Templin, PT, DPT, GCS and
Owner at *HouseFit*, St. Louis, MO

CONTENTS

A LETTER FROM CHRISTINE

Dear all,

I invite you to step into my life for a brief moment:
"MOMMY!"
It's another morning where I'm woken up by the screams of children.
"Mommy... I'm hungry!"
Rolling over, I glance at the clock. As I throw off the covers and slide out of bed, I think I'm just a tired mom trying to raise two kids, both under five, while running two businesses that I started myself. Who wouldn't be tired?
My kids are bounding down the stairs already declaring their breakfast desires; cereal for my daughter and "ba-ba", or bottle, for my son. He's 18 months old and I haven't had the time or energy to wean the morning bottle. I stop, breathe, and get moving.
My daughter fires up her iPad and YouTube blares a few decibels too loud. My son cuddles into my lap, holding his stuffed dog and favorite blanket. While he's drinking his bottle is one of the few times one might find him sitting still during the day. Otherwise, though, he's high energy, dunking balls, throwing balls, dribbling balls, and copying every move his sister makes.
In these precious moments, we all sit huddled together on the sofa. This sofa has seen a lot of family history, and it also happens to be the most comfortable sofa we've ever had. For those reasons, we keep it – despite the fact it is a complete eyesore. The drop cloth cover that I made is pulling off in multiple places. There are children's

red marker lines all over one of the cushions. It's so old it probably smells. But, I don't notice it anymore.

This sofa was given to us by my in-laws. In fact, my husband grew up with it in his family living room. It's long past its prime, but it still wins as the most comfortable sofa ever. And I should know: I've spent a whole lot of time on this sofa.

Yes. This sofa was where I spent 3 months laying on my side while on bedrest with my daughter. Later, I spent another 3 months in the same position with my son. All in all, you can say this sofa and I have "bonded." More on that later, though.

For now, while we all snuggle on our favorite sofa, I take a moment to pull out my phone and look at my day. Mondays are always busy. I scan the calendar before pulling up my two work emails to check on both my businesses. As usual, there are so many emails it can get overwhelming; I quickly try to delete anything that can be moved to the trash. As I scan, I also look for ones that need to be taken care of as soon as possible. Within seconds, my eyes find it; I have two new inquiries from my physical therapy clinic's website.

I can't help but smile. While I was sleeping last night, my physical therapy clinic's website was working for me, getting my message out to the people who have problems I can help with. And, because of that, I now have two hot leads to follow-up with today – I can start the process of securing a patient.

My point is this: I now see how the months I spent laying on this exact sofa, the one that transformed me into a business owner, and then again into a multi-business owner, were not wasted. In fact, they completely changed my life.

Starting a business is never easy... running a business is even harder, and maintaining a steady source of income, of new patients, of leads is, well, almost impossible. Right?

I used to think so too, but it doesn't have to be. I can honestly say that, as a mother of two children and the owner of two successful business, you CAN achieve your dreams of financial and personal success.

I wrote this book for you. It's a book about success, about failures, about the will to overcome adversity. It's also a book about the immense potential of your business's website, not only for your bank account, but for your personal life. This is a book meant to reach you directly, to get you excited about the future, to give you the tools to take charge of your business via your website. I know you can do it.

In the following pages, I outline exactly how achieving financial freedom is closer than you think. Join me as we uncover the secrets of a successful website and your key to realizing the dreams you've always had for your business.

I look forward this journey together, and I wish you every success.

Let's get started!

INTRODUCTION

Most physical therapy websites are a waste of money. Instead of bringing more patients and more profit into the business, they sit on the internet like a pretty online resume, a business card, or even worse, they actually scare people away from the business.

The gut reaction of most physical therapy business owners is to ignore the fact their website isn't working and hustle to get referrals by begging other sources, such as doctors, gyms, and yoga/Pilates studios. Even scarier, some owners depend solely on former clients and word of mouth for their business to survive. These tactics may work for a while, but at a certain point the business will get stuck and be unable to grow any more.

It's particularly devastating when PT business owners realize that the website that they've spent thousands of dollars (or thousands of hours) on doesn't work. It's even more outrageous that so many business owners are content to live with such a dysfunctional website. How are you going to break free from being a slave to all of your referral sources *without* a working website you can use to bring you more new patients to your business *on your own*?

Understanding that your website is failing you and your business isn't easy. I'm here to share my story so that YOUR realization happens sooner rather than later. If you're not making money from your PT clinic's website, something is wrong.

It's devastating when your business isn't growing and the phones aren't ringing. In that silence we're not sure where the next new patient is going to come from. The doubt starts to creep in, and we wonder whether we're good enough or ever will be.

And the worst part is that the doubt doesn't cease because we have advanced degrees and spent years in school learning how to treat patients. When your business is struggling, you wonder, what actually went wrong? Is it possible to fix? What needs to be fixed? You start to wonder if you are the actual problem... In these dark places, we dread having to go back to working for someone else as a *staff* physical therapist.

Can you relate? Do you see yourself in this scenario? Is your business failing? Are the phones not ringing and the patients not coming in? And are you starting to believe YOU'RE the problem?

There's hope. I want to tell you something that might change your life: the problem isn't *you* or the business you worked so hard to build. In fact, what if the problem is simpler than that? What if the problem is the way your physical therapy business is positioned online?

Not convinced?

The web developers and big physical therapy website companies we hire to build our websites are experts in technology and Search Engine Optimization (SEO), but how many of them can actually tell you what physical therapy *really* is? How many of them have experienced *cash-paid* or *out-of-network* physical therapy themselves?

These companies are happy to take our money, build us a pretty website, optimize our SEO, and maybe even make a newsletter for us, but they do all this REGARDLESS of whether or not those things actually bring you more new patients or grow your business.

Something is seriously wrong. You're spending thousands of dollars on a website that isn't even breaking even. You're not getting new patients, you're not getting calls, you're website's not converting, and there are no feet coming through your clinic doors!

The vast majority of physical therapy websites don't actually attract new patients. **We've missed the mark.**

It's actually possible to have a physical therapy website that does grow your business and finally bring in more new patients. I know *this* because I'm now working with hundreds of physical therapy business owners just like you around the world; I'm helping them transform their websites into patient-generating machines.

Making changes and inspecting your website isn't necessarily easy. I know. But the change needs to be made, and it needs to be made RIGHT NOW. I understand your hesitation, and I definitely understand your fear. But if I could make this change, so can you.

• • •

I was once in the same position: I was faced with a website that wasn't working and the realization that something needed to change. My first website, which I spent months building, was a complete flop and attracted ZERO new patients the first year it existed. Honestly. I had NO new patients being generated online. I had almost no cash flow, fewer patients, and absolutely no idea what to do.

The frustration of having a flat-lined cash physical therapy practice almost drove me back into the world of working for someone else. But, instead of giving in and giving up my dream, I hunkered down and decided that if other businesses could get new clients off the internet, I could too.

This led me to create my *PT Website Secrets™ System*. I created this framework to successfully transform my own website, one which is designed to attract, find, and secure new patients. Instantaneously, I had new patients, new leads, and a new life. Why? Because I knew that my website would predictably bring in new patients.

The success of my website was witnessed by my peers, and, after noticing my success, I had dozens of other physical therapists asking me to help them do the same thing for their small businesses. To date, I have taught this system to *over one hundred physical therapists* across the globe.

That's 100+ successful websites, 100+ happy PT owners, 100+ profitable business, and 100+ times I made a difference and helped more people who needed physical therapy get into a physical therapist's office.

Once my clients get their website transformed, they experience incredible results. Why? Because after learning the *PT Website Secrets*™ *System*, they know **what** their website is for, they know **who** their website is for, and they know **how** to actually sell physical therapy. Yes, that's right. They KNOW HOW TO MAKE THEIR WEBSITE WORK FOR THEM.

At *PT Website Secrets*™ we've had clients get a 900% return on their investment in only two weeks. *PT Website Secrets*™ is so powerful that we've seen other companies add over $40,000 to their yearly bottom line by adding one button to their website. And all of this was achieved by getting the message and the design of their websites right!

The *PT Website Secrets*™ *System* has been incredibly effective not just for cash-based practices but also for out-of-network, hybrid, and even insurance-based clinics. This system makes it possible for physical therapy clinics to generate new patients with their online presence. Yet, despite this immense potential, too many clinics aren't taking advantage of this opportunity. What are you waiting for? Perhaps you haven't asked yourself these questions yet:

1. **How many new patients is your clinic missing out on because you don't have your website nailed?**
2. **How much money have you lost?**
3. **Even more importantly, how many more people could you be impacting in your community? How many could you be saving from things like unnecessary surgery, large numbers of expensive visits to the physician, and dangerous painkillers and injections?**

If you don't know the answers to these questions, or you've been too afraid to be honest with yourself about them, I challenge you to ask yourself this: **what are you waiting for?**

What you're above to discover in this book is a system that will lay out the formula for getting a website that brings in more patients and more profit. You'll see exactly how you can set up a website so that it's your "hardest working employee."

I'm about to take you from confused, stressed, and tempted to throw your computer out the window (please don't) to enjoying the process of building your online presence. It's time to really show the world what you can do for them as a physical therapist. **Now, let the book begin...**

1

WHY MOST WEBSITES ARE MONEY PITS (INSTEAD OF MONEY MAKERS)

My first website was a complete flop. Yes, that's right. It was an absolute disaster. In fact, it was the exact opposite of what I as a PT owner wanted from my website. What I wanted was my "hardest working employee," one that generates new patient leads for me each night while I'm sleeping, or when I'm at the park with my kids, or even while I'm vacationing at the beach. What I got was... well, a staff member who's off sick 6/7 days a week. In other words, it was the exact opposite of my current website! In fact, my first website wasn't bad, it was an utter failure.

It's not unusual for a new PT business owner to attempt the construction of their own website. Some undertake the task because they don't know there are other options out there. Others do it because they feel that they're so strapped for cash they can't afford to invest in their website (not realizing that if they get the right one, they could increase their investment tenfold!). In my case, however, I attempted my first website because I was forced to.

Although I considered myself to be somewhat tech-savvy, when I first thought about creating a website for my new cash practice, I certainly didn't think I'd do it myself. I don't have any computer coding skills, but, like many millennials, I perfected the art of computer multitasking as a teenager. Once the internet became something accessible to the masses, albeit via dial tone, I was your typical teenager: I spent hours having conversations on AOL's AIM, downloading music, and doing goodness knows what. *YouTube* and *Netflix* weren't even around back then. All I remember is having fifteen or more conversations at a time while my parents marveled at how I could keep track of it all.

In other words, at the outset my computer skills were fine, but they weren't anything special. I wasn't writing computer programs or inventing new online games like some kids these days. So, when I became a business owner and needed a website, I didn't think I'd be the one to do it.

In my mind, the logical next step was to look around at all the big companies that advertise themselves as being experts in physical therapy websites and marketing. I wanted something that would work, and I knew that my physical therapy marketing knowledge was zero to none.

I spent time talking to all the well-known companies on the market. I watched their webinars, attended free demos, and did my research. They seemed to have a lot of happy customers, and they seemed to know a lot about stuff I was clueless about such as SEO, page rankings, and content creation. To be honest, they knew how to make flashy and professional looking websites.

But I remember being a little surprised by their own marketing strategies. Not having been exposed to that sort of thing before, I assumed that what their websites touted – features such as "professional design," "support throughout the process," and "stand out from the crowd" – was the right thing. Naturally, I went ahead thinking that this is what it meant to have a successful physical therapy website: a flashy logo, professional design, and content about how unique my practice was. But then I started to wonder...'if that's all it takes to get new patients, then maybe I could build a website like that myself.

As luck would have it life made the decision for me. I was suddenly put on activity restrictions while pregnant with my second child. The reality of ZERO income for six months forced the decision. In my mind, I couldn't afford to do anything but make my own website. While this seemed like the best short-term decision to keep the bank account above zero, little did I know how much money this decision would cost my family and my business in the long run. In fact, I had no idea how terribly wrong I went with my first website.

MISTAKE #1 – WHY MY FIRST WEBSITE FLOPPED

LOOK BEYOND THE HOMEPAGE

Whether you're building your own website or have hired someone to do it for you, the natural instinct is to go look for inspiration from other physical therapy websites. When I was forced to build my own website, I immediately needed inspiration.

What did I do? I started looking at the websites of other successful clinics in town. I assumed that they must know how to make patient-generating websites since they *appeared* to be thriving businesses which were seeing lots of patients. One by one, I poured through the pages of these glamorous websites. I would take notes on the parts that I liked, and I omitted any elements that weren't my style. Taking inspiration from these clinics seemed like the most logical step. They appeared to have booming businesses, so shouldn't their websites be successful?

What I failed to consider when looking at other physical therapy websites is that I had no idea whether or not these businesses were actually getting new patients from the Internet. While their weekly schedules might have been full, I later discovered that most physical therapy clinics do NOT get many new patients from online platforms. Instead, they rely on "hustle-style" marketing.

And where does this hustle-style marketing become most obvious? For the insurance-based clinics it is, of course, in doctors rooms. Sometimes they even have their own doctors employed by the same company in order to have a steady stream of patients. Other clinic owners – those who do not have the luxury of having their own doctors – work themselves very hard by visiting gyms, yoga and Pilates studios, and *CrossFit* boxes. Others hold workshops and speak at events. And then, of course, you always see the clinics that buy a tent at a local health fair. All of these techniques meld together to become what I now call "hustle-style marketing" (also known as marketing that's NOT possible when you're pregnant and on bedrest!).

The harsh reality was that the websites I drew inspiration from didn't actually use their online presence to generate significant amounts of new patients. They were still doing lots of hustle-style marketing in order to grow their business. I had taken my inspiration from the wrong people.

MISTAKE #2 – WHY MY FIRST WEBSITE FLOPPED

PRETTY ISN'T ALWAYS BEST

The websites that I admired and studied before making my first site had one obvious element in common: they had **tremendous visual appeal**.

Let's be honest – when it comes to picking things in life, looks matter. Whether it's the fruit in the grocery store or the person you want to marry, it's hard to deny that we are persuaded by visual appeal.

Since I work with websites every day, I am frequently targeted online by ads from other website companies, and some days I find it hard not to laugh out loud. Why? Because, if you look around, a lot of website marketing will tell you that if your website isn't sleek, sexy, and professional then it won't be effective. I want to let you in on a big secret – **this is a complete lie**.

Yet, at the beginning I bought into this lie wholeheartedly. I spent hours agonizing over the perfect pictures for my *Homepage*.

I selected pictures that I thought my patients would want to see, ones that might envision a patient's life after physical therapy. I considered people exercising on the beach, running in the sunset, and doing yoga by the lake. They all made "getting active again" look so appealing. Isn't that what my patients wanted to see?

After I finally settled on a picture of a woman walking into the sunset, I turned to designing my logo. I went back and forth with an online designer, agonizing over the right color blue, the right size, and the right feel. I wanted it to be perfect.

Little did I know it at the time, but pretty pictures and logos are not what makes your physical therapy website successful, and they certainly don't help you grow your business.

In fact, the scary thing is that pictures may actually be deterring website visitors from calling your practice. Pictures are very powerful, but they are also very subjective and can be interpreted in many ways, something we'll talk more about in Chapter 7.

MISTAKE #3 – WHY MY FIRST WEBSITE FLOPPED

NOT WHO ARE *YOU*, WHO IS YOUR PATIENT?

By most standards, I started my cash practice very early in my career: only three years after graduating from physical therapy school. To make matters worse, I looked young and I knew it. One of my patients jokingly introduces me to everyone as his "16 year old physical therapist," this despite the fact I've been married nine years and have two kids at the time of this writing. I don't take it too personally (as I'm sure I'll like this if it lasts till I'm 40), but I thought I was at a huge disadvantage when it came to marketing because I looked so young.

On my website I was determined to show that, despite my age and appearance, I was highly qualified and that my services were worth paying for out-of-pocket. One of the main things I tried to do was to prove my worth on my website. Here, I touted all of my accomplishments, extra training, and credentials. I thought that if people saw **how much I had done, then maybe they would trust me** despite my youth.

Hence, my biography was full of my accomplishments. I wanted everyone to know that I went to a great undergraduate program at *UNC-Chapel Hill* and that I went to a well-known physical therapy school, the *Medical University of South Carolina*. I wanted them to know about all my accomplishments, including that I was named a Presidential Scholar, and that I sat and took my 'Performance Enhancement Specialist' certification from the *National Academy of Sports Medicine* while I was in PT school. And, of course, I wanted to highlight my newly acquired Professional Yoga Therapist certification which was an extensive amount of coursework. I pretty much thought that my resume should speak for itself.

The real mistake here was thinking that my PT business website was actually supposed to be about me, and that, in fact, this couldn't be farther from the truth! Because guess what? My website shouldn't be about me... it should always be about the patient!

It turns out that patients are as egocentric as we are. Sure, they want to know that you are qualified to provide healthcare, but really all they want to know that you can help them. They really don't understand all the fancy letters behind your name. All those special treatment techniques seem like a foreign language to them.

Patients don't care who gets them better – whether it be a physical therapist, massage therapist, personal trainer, chiropractor or even a physician. They don't care about where you went to school. They want to get better and get back to doing whatever it is they love. It's that simple.

As much as I thought my website was about me, it turns out it should be about my patients.

MISTAKE #4 – WHY MY FIRST WEBSITE FLOPPED

THE MYTH OF "BOOK NOW"

When I was looking around at other physical therapy websites, it became apparent that everyone was asking people to either "book now" or "call now for an appointment." Sometimes you would see this up in the header of a website, and other times it would be part of a large and flashy photo or slideshow scrolling across the top of the homepage. Since so many clinics had this on their website, I assumed (wrongly) that having a "book now" or "call now" button must work in getting website visitors to become patients.

On my *Homepage*, therefore, I carefully crafted a headline and button to overlay on my professional "walking into the sunset" photo. Here's what it looked like:

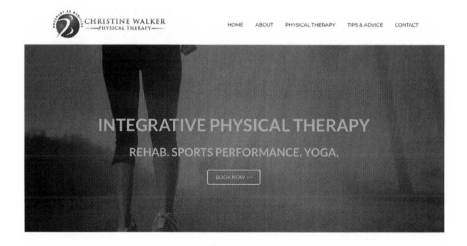

As you can see, I thought people would be interested in:

- Integrative Physical Therapy
- Rehab. Yoga. Performance.
- BOOK NOW!

My thought process was this: a website visitor will see an attractive woman walking into the sunset, and simultaneously, they'll know from my headline that I'm a holistic and integrative clinic that will provide a unique healthcare experience. Thus, (in an instant) they will want to call and talk to me!

What I failed to consider is that most people who land on a website aren't ready to "book now." In fact, they're just starting to check you out and get to know you. They still don't trust you. They are shopping around.

Think about your own behavior. When you're looking to buy a new television, do you go on *Amazon* and buy the first one that pops up in your search results? Of course not! Instead, you look at the specifications, you read reviews, and you look at different stores to find the best deal.

People are doing the same thing with your physical therapy website. They're finding you, looking around, and then comparing you to other options in town. In fact, most people won't be ready to commit to an appointment until they have had multiple points of contact with your clinic, whether that's by email, advertisement, phone calls, or other forms of personal interaction.

All the "book now" and "call now" buttons do is rush the relationship and scare away potential patients. My attempts at encouraging people to do business with me were like asking someone to go from *dating* to *married* without them ever meeting in person!

MISTAKE #5 – WHY MY FIRST WEBSITE FLOPPED

TOO MUCH INFORMATION

Since I was a cash practice, and did not take insurance like most physical therapy clinics, I felt like I needed to justify my decision on my website. I was so uncomfortable with the *"do you take my insurance"* question that I naively thought I could get that conversation over with online. In theory, this sounded like a good idea. I wanted my potential clients to be aware of how I was different, and *why*.

I dedicated an entire page to answering questions about my physical therapy clinic. It was titled "FAQ," and on it I addressed why I was "out-of-network" with insurance companies and what that meant for the consumer. I had worksheets explaining how the patient could call their insurance companies and understand their benefits. I also made sure to talk about what benefits a patient would receive because of my out-of-network status. Worst of all, I actually listed the prices of my services.

Little did I know that this page was probably one of the biggest reasons for my business' stifled growth. Why? Because most people don't understand what physical therapy is, **and they don't buy things they don't understand**. That also means they definitely don't understand the differences between two different physical therapy clinics and are therefore very likely to pick the cheapest one.

Remember, our natural tendency is to think that many things we purchase are equal. What's the difference between two televisions? Maybe a slight picture quality difference, but will you really notice once you get the television home? The same goes for picking which hotel you want to stay at when you're on vacation. How many times have you been willing to stay in a Three-Star hotel to save some money instead of staying at the Five-Star resort?

People hardly understand the difference between physical therapists, chiropractors, and even personal trainers, so how can we expect them to understand the different benefits between an in-network and out-of-network clinic? It's an argument you're going to lose.

What's more, if you put your price on your website, then you've already lost the game before getting a chance to play. How many times do you quickly look up a service and then dismiss it because of the price? I know that's the first thing I look for when scanning a new product or service.

PUBLISHED

Despite all these mistakes (which I didn't know about at the time), I still remember the relief I felt when I hit the publish button for the first time. After weeks of researching, editing, and getting things "just right," I finally had a website for my new cash physical therapy practice. I was proud that I had actually figured out how to use a drag and drop website builder to build a professional-looking website for my new cash practice.

So, I did what anyone else might do: I sent an email to all my friends and family announcing my new business venture and inviting them to take a look at my website.

The response was overwhelming. The compliments poured in. Everyone was so impressed I had made my own website and that it looked very professional. The truth is, I thought I had it right. I talked about how different I was from every other PT in Charlotte, how I provided one-on-one care, how I approached physical therapy from a holistic premise. Now that my business was well represented on the Internet, what would stop me from succeeding?

WHAT HAPPENS WHEN CLINICS DON'T HAVE AN EFFECTIVE WEBSITE?

One year after building my own PT website, reality set in. My business was seeing less than five patients a week and they were all from word of mouth referrals and hustle-style marketing. Every night I would lie awake wondering when the next new patient would come in, or if I would be able to pay not only my business expenses for the month, but also the family bills.

Despite my highly acclaimed website, no one had ever called me from it asking to book an appointment. I tried running advertisements, putting out business cards, visiting with *CrossFit* gyms and yoga studios, but I still didn't get any new patients from my website. The online analytics revealed that plenty of people were visiting my website, but they would look around for a little while and then leave. Why didn't they call? Why didn't they email me? Didn't they realize that I could help them?

I started to doubt whether or not I was really capable of owning my own physical therapy practice. Maybe I didn't have what it takes. Maybe I would have to go back to working full-time for someone else, missing out on important things with my family, and being stuck as a slave to the insurance companies.

After one year of waiting for the phone to ring, I decided something had to be done. It was time to either close up my practice OR to take a serious look at why my physical therapy practice wasn't growing and why my website wasn't working. Thankfully, I chose the latter.

• • •

If you're currently in the same situation, feeling hopeless, afraid, and worried, then read on. I want to change your life by changing your website! *PT Website Secrets*™ is here to help – no more failing websites, silent phones, and empty clinics. Things need to change and we're going to do it together! Let's go!

2

FROM BROKE & ON BEDREST TO BUSINESS OWNER: COULD THIS WORK FOR YOU TOO?

BUSINESS OWNER BY ACCIDENT

My story is unconventional in some ways, but in the fundamental truths of it, I believe all PT owners go through the same fundamental struggles I went through. The doubt, the anxiety, the worry... I had it all. In fact, the *ups* and *downs* of my story all culminate in one overarching truth....my cash practice started by accident. Yes – that's right. The thought of owning my own cash practice dawned on me at the most unexpected time. Who starts a cash practice (without knowing what you're doing) between having two kids? Me, apparently.

If you had asked me, as a youngster, if I considered myself entrepreneurial, the words "NO" would have been out of my mouth in a heartbeat. I was scared to death of the idea of running my own business. I wasn't afraid of the challenge, the money, or the hard work... I was afraid of being afraid! Yes, as a first-born child and obsessive rule-follower, the idea of the Internal Revenue Service (IRS) coming after me for messing something up was terrifying.

Rules and regulations bound me to thinking inside the box for a long time.

Despite this, it's clear on reflection that I had an entrepreneur's spirit from an early age. I took advantage of my talents in both soccer and springboard diving and used them to teach others. Moreover, as a teenager I held my own training camps for young, female soccer players, and a few years later I even started a springboard diving program for kids at my local pool.

Ultimately, the first time I really considered owning my own physical therapy practice was on my first clinical rotation.

MY FIRST CLINICAL ROTATION RUINED ME

I was so full of excitement for my first clinical rotation. Like many other physical therapy students, I was sick of sitting in the classroom and was itching to work with real patients. I was especially excited because my first clinic assignment was in outpatient orthopedics at *Imagine Physical Therapy - Daniel Island* in Charleston, South Carolina. I was passionate about orthopedics and believed that my calling was to work with athletes.

I started my rotation under the supervision of Kris Winders, a former college basketball player who towered over me at 6' 8". I still remember the moment we spoke on the phone before my first day. Immediately, I knew there was something different about this physical therapy clinic. First off, he explained how the clinic took a two hour break at lunchtime in order to allow their employees to exercise. That was a huge surprise, as few companies value their employees enough to give them a break to take care of themselves.

If I thought that was unique, the next difference completely blew me away. Kris asked me if I was comfortable being at the office at 8:00 AM in order to have Bible study and pray for the patients coming in that day. He assured me that students were not required to participate but were invited to join. I remember feeling shocked, excited, and overwhelmed with gratitude to be able to see how a Christian-run business operated.

Based on the Bible verse (Ephesians 3:20) which reads, "... more than we can ever ask or imagine," *Imagine Physical Therapy* clinic lives up to its name. My time there opened my eyes to a world so different from the 'mill-like' clinics that dot the country, and I can honestly say my experience there *ruined* everything I ever thought I knew about physical therapy.

I found myself in a world where physical therapists spent lots of one-on-one time with their patients, where everyone knew not only their patients names, but also the names of all the patient's family members. Laughter and stories constantly filled the 2-room clinic. From the outside you would not have guessed it was a place where people with injuries conjugated.

Kris had created a physical therapy clinic that was all about the experience, and yet he was still turning a profit even as an insurance-based business.[1] Being there was unlike anything I could have hoped for: seeing others receive treatment like THAT in an insurance based clinic in the US is almost unheard of. From the moment I arrived, I knew that this was how I wanted to practice physical therapy.

THERE'S MORE THAN ONE WAY TO MAKE A PROFIT

The biggest lesson I learned during my time in Charleston is that the success of a physical therapy business is not based on meeting a patient's functional goals, or over scheduling therapists in order to maximize profit. Now, I don't have anything against making a profit, I just don't like to do it at the expense of the people who keep me in business – my patients. Instead, success comes from achieving the outcome that the patient wants.

The most amazing thing I learned is that patients don't care as much about "getting out of pain" as you would think. Instead, they

---

1 Kris has since moved back to his hometown of Lexington, KY and founded the highly successful *BBN Physical Therapy*. You'll hear more of his story later in the book!

care more about the journey or experience that gets them back to doing the things they love. So what do patients actually love?

The 40 year-old husband who works in corporate America loves to escape the house and kids on the weekend and play a relaxing round of golf with his buddies.

The youth athlete doesn't want to miss a game, or even a practice if possible, because it's where he gets both his athletic and social fulfillment, taking the stress off of being a teenager.

The grandmother wants to be mobile and free from painkillers so that she can take care of her grandchildren. Why? Because they give her a second chance to "get things right" and being with the grandchildren makes her feel youthful again.

There are so many other stories...

These people don't care about pain. They care about their experiences. This is a concept we'll keep coming back to throughout the book.

THERE AREN'T THAT MANY *IMAGINE PHYSICAL THERAPY* CLINICS OUT THERE

A year and a half later, after finishing all four of my clinic rotations, reality set in. I was not going to work for a mill-like clinic that is overbooked, understaffed, and not patient-orientated. There was no way I could ever go work full-time in a standard outpatient physical therapy clinic. Period. So what was I going to do with my career?

Well, my determination was put on the back burner, I guess you could say. I had my dreams, but life got in the way. I didn't let go of my hopes, but I didn't grab them then and there. Thus, following graduation I was faced with the reality of taking a job in a "PT factory" or going after my second passion, pediatrics.

It was a fairly easy choice. I started in outpatient pediatrics, yet I found myself itching to be in a different setting. Coming from a family of physicians I was really comfortable in the hospital and so I took a PRN job working in acute care. While it wasn't strictly pediatrics or orthopedics, I loved the fact that no day ever looked the same and that my schedule was constantly changing.

Shortly after transitioning to the acute care setting, my husband and I decided to try to get pregnant. Eight months after graduating PT school, I eagerly surprised my husband with the news that we were expecting our first child. We were both so excited, but the truth is you never know what's going to happen when you have kids. We entered the pregnancy with a lot of hope, but little did we know things were about to change really fast.

"I CAN'T TAKE ANOTHER STEP"

Everything was normal – I was working as usual and I was as enthusiastic as ever. But everything changed on Father's Day weekend in 2013. I had been back to D.C. to visit my dad, and while there we did an unusually large amount of walking, after working all week in the hospital. Never having had any problems during my pregnancy with walking, I didn't think much of it.

On Saturday night, everything started going wrong. While walking to the theater to watch a comedy group, *The Capitol Steps*, I suddenly couldn't walk another step. My father, being the supportive figure he has always been – in fact, he's a doctor – urged me to go to the hospital immediately. I refused, however, stating that I only needed to rest. Truth be told, I was so confused about the situation and the suddenness of it that I hardly had a moment to register the severity. So, having explained that I just needed to rest, we took a bike taxi the final 3 blocks to the show.

My thought process at the time was that I had worked 40 hours at the hospital, and not only that, I had walked countless miles over the last couple of days. In my mind rest was all I needed, but nevertheless I called my midwife when I returned home. I had a feeling that whatever it was, it needed to be checked out.

My midwife, Jan, wanted me to come in immediately. That was a little nerve-wrecking, but at the time I still didn't realize the severity of the situation. So, as I waited for Jan to explain what was going on, the anxiety and fear grew within me.

Having children is surrendering to something greater than yourself. You love so intensely and completely that the idea of losing your child is an unimaginable grief. All I could do was stare at the 3D ultrasound image of my daughter's face and think, "will I ever see *you* alive?" I sat in the waiting room, tears spilling down my face silently. All I could do was pray for strength, courage, and peace for whatever the outcome would be.

THE REALITY OF BEDREST

The midwife explained that the pain I was feeling was my body making preparations to deliver. Since I was only 23 weeks pregnant, this was a serious issue. Only 20-35% of babies born at 23 weeks survive, and the babies that do survive typically have life-long complications. My heart absolutely sank, but it was also in that moment when I realized that my husband's and my sole mission was to protect our unborn daughter. I worked at a pediatric hospital. I knew the odds. I was going to do everything possible to give my daughter the best shot at surviving. So, at 23 weeks pregnant, I went on bedrest: I was only allowed off the couch for 5 minutes every hour.

For 13 weeks I lay on my side on that old sofa with my faithful Labrador retriever, Penny, at my feet. My emotions fluctuated from scared, to hopeful, to distraught – I was literally stuck on a couch for 3 months. Ultimately, though, I came to find a sense of peace and purpose.

On October 15, 2013, our daughter Virginia made a very rapid appearance into the world. I guess one of the advantages of my pregnancy complications was a quick delivery! Virginia is a blessing, and having her with us today is a constant reminder of the amazing gift of life and of God's faithfulness. I try to remember that on a daily basis – when I work with patients, with clients, and with my family. Life is precious, and it is a privilege and blessing that I get to work alongside others to help people fight through their medical struggles.

Once Virginia was born, I thought the worst of my pregnancy would be over and life would start to return to "normal" – as normal as you can get for first time parents having a newborn. At least I was allowed to get off the sofa now! The only problem was... I couldn't.

Gifts often come in the most unlikely of ways. Let me explain. My daughter brought such an intense light to my life that, and quite apart from blessing my family with her presence, she also opened the door to an unexplored and little confronted part of myself. The arrival of my daughter coincided with one of the hardest times in my life: a time without which I would not be who I am today. It took the birth of my first child to usher me into one of the biggest challenges I have ever faced, the outcome of which, through intense suffering, endurance, and heartache, resulted in not only personal growth, but business success.

I COULDN'T GET OUT OF BED

Following my daughter's birth, I found myself falling further and further into a little-known condition called *postpartum obsessive compulsive disorder (OCD)*. Unlike the slightly more common *postpartum depression*, postpartum OCD is hardly ever spoken about. I had very little idea what that was, let alone how to face it.

If you look up the symptoms of postpartum OCD, they're pretty scary. You have overwhelming thoughts surrounding the safety and security of your baby. You excessively worry about the baby dying in her sleep, and, as it gets worse, you actually start thinking about your baby dying because of your own doing. Ultimately, I started to be afraid of being around my daughter, thinking that I might harm her. Later still, I started to worry someone would take her away from me because I might be a danger to her.

Before I was diagnosed with the condition and understood it clearly, I felt as though I was sinking into a mental breakdown.

I couldn't sleep. I wasn't eating. I couldn't even get out of bed. I couldn't talk to anyone without withdrawing and shutting down emotionally. Clearly, I couldn't go back to work.

You can imagine that, as a new mother and the caretaker of my beautiful baby girl, thoughts of harming her, fears for her safety, and even frightening and persistent depression and OCD tendencies, was overwhelming. I was questioning my very ability to be a good mother. I felt as though I was failing. The guilt nearly broke me, and after a while I lost my appetite completely, stopped socializing, and lay in bed all day in the hope that the feelings of guilt, anxiety, and depression might go away.

WHY SHARE THIS?

You might be wondering why I'm sharing all this with you. At the time, I couldn't talk about it. In fact, I was extremely embarrassed to mention that this was going on. I bought into the lie that it was something I could control on my own. As the years have passed, I've come to realize that by *not* talking about this time in my life I'm only perpetuating the problem: most families don't want to discuss experiences like mental breakdowns. This book gives me an opportunity to turn my harrowing experience into something positive; it gives me the space to change that past hurt into something usable and valuable for you right now.

WHEN WILL THIS END?

During that time in my life, those awful thoughts didn't go away. Instead, they consumed me. I no longer went to work and I was paralyzed with fear. I was losing myself. It was at this point that my husband and father, two men I greatly admire, stepped in.

I remember it all happened one weekend – a weekend unremarkable in the fact that I was, once again, confined to my bed in a state of mental unrest. My husband told me that whatever was going on was "not normal" and that I needed to get help. That we couldn't keep going on "like this." My dad said essentially said the same thing. He said that at three months postpartum I should not be holed up in bed. Something had to be done.

It was at that moment, not knowing the exact cause of what I was going through or how much longer it would last, that I agreed. If something didn't change I would lose not only my happiness but everything that made me who I am.

OUT OF THE DARKNESS

I was immediately placed into a Christian counseling program; I also saw a psychiatrist and was prescribed medication. After a time filled with determination, love, heartache, and many defeats, I started feeling a lot better. Recovery isn't an easy thing, but what is important to realize – and for those of you who might be in a similar situation or know someone going through this – it's a **condition** and **there is help**. You can overcome it.

My battle with postpartum OCD opened a doorway for me. I came to explore not only my current fears but also my past struggles with fear. Remember how I mentioned my entrepreneurial nature, one which I never pursued because of fear? Well, if I hadn't had my daughter I never would have confronted some of the deepest fears in myself, and I never would have gained the success I have today. The old me would not have ever started even one real business. The new me has now started two.

After I felt better I started to get the itch to recreate, or capture, a part of the experience I had at *Imagine Physical Therapy*.

The only question is, why hadn't I done it before?

The truth is that, to some degree, I had been prone to that fearful, obsessive mindset my entire life. It took a complete crash in order to see what was really holding me back from realizing my dreams and serving the people who I've been called to help. I had not reached my personal or financial goals. Why not? Because my mind had been holding me back! And think, if it weren't for my experience after giving birth to my daughter, this book wouldn't even exist.

In that moment, everything changed. I couldn't go back to working as a staff physical therapist, so I hit the ground running, making significant changes in my life. I stopped obsessing and started DOING.

I now run two profitable businesses. And, if it weren't for my first pregnancy and the transformations that followed it, I wouldn't be here, let alone be a successful, ambitious, excited UNAFRAID entrepreneur. I would be working in a job only for the sake of making money; I would be unhappy and afraid. The type of life changing transformation I underwent is what I hope you will experience in your own life – to be unafraid of realizing your dreams no matter how hard it might seem at times.

CASH PRACTICE BEGINNINGS

My cash practice started small, in fact, it started as a mobile practice that went to people's homes. For a while I only had one patient, once a week, and I spent my extra hours filling in at the local children's hospital. It didn't take long before I fell in love with having control over my own schedule. The flexibility it afforded me as a mom who wanted to spend some time caring for her daughter was incredible.

Never let anyone tell you that managing your own time is overrated – it isn't, and I hope this book will give you the courage and tools to make it happen. I loved every moment of having my own practice, and I wanted to learn as much as I could.

During its first year my cash practice slowly picked up patients from my hustle-style marketing and word of mouth efforts. Remember hustle-style marketing from Chapter 1? Well, I was doing it day in and day out. Yet, despite a *whole lot of hustling, my* business enjoyed only minor *benefits*. During this time, my pretty website was busy sitting online, getting some traffic, but not resulting in any calls. That professional-looking website was not getting me the business I needed to quit my other job!

Also at this time, my husband and I were contemplating another child. After all, doesn't everyone decide to go have a new baby after starting a new business? Just kidding... it was a scary thought. My first pregnancy and postpartum was complicated, to say the least. While pregnant with my daughter I was put on three months of strict bedrest. Then, after my daughter's birth, I suffered from postpartum OCD, which had almost taken away my joy in life, family, and work completely.

As could be expected, I was anxious about having another baby. Nonetheless, my husband and I had a strong desire for our little girl to have a sibling, and we'd always wanted more than one child.

Having another baby was a tough decision for both of us. My husband knew he might be thrown back into "taking care of everything," but now "everything" included a two year old girl. For me, I had come so far from the depths of postpartum OCD to being a new business owner. Through faith, though, my husband and I decided to be courageous and try having another child. And the desires of our hearts were met.

IT'S HAPPENING AGAIN

I joyfully fell pregnant with my second child only to find out early on the same complications that put me on bedrest with my daughter were happening again. Though overwhelmed with happiness about having a son, my business momentum was shot. My cash practice was going to be put to the test because as a PT I was out of commission for a while, and, let's be honest, how could a solo PT practice survive without a physical therapist?

The reality of all this set in at around the 26th week of my pregnancy. It dawned on me that I would have to restrict my activity levels again, which consequently meant that I couldn't do the hustle-style marketing that kept my business alive and running... and me on my feet all day! I was faced with the choice to either shut down my practice or find a way to ensure its survival through a financial drought of bedrest and maternity leave.

Here's the thing... the easy choice would have been to give up on my dream of owning my own practice, of being able to treat the patients I loved in the way I know they should be treated, and of being truly satisfied in my profession. But I wasn't going to let my dreams go; I had to make it work. I had to do it not only for me but for my family and my patients. So, instead of letting my circumstances get me down, I realized that I needed to utilize the time I'd been given wisely. My family needed me. My private patients needed me. *I* needed me.

Once the decision to overcome this obstacle was made, I had a lot of time to sit around and reflect on my business. Soon, it became clear I was on the cusp of a crucial decision. Did I want my cash practice to be something that I dabbled in for fun on the side? Or did I want to take my business seriously and change the trajectory of my career as a physical therapist?

This decision is one that, I feel, each and every one of you has had to make, is in the process of making, or will still need to make. As physical therapists wanting to start your own practices, this is one of the most important choices we will ever make, and trust me, I know it isn't easy.

As I weighed the decision, I turned to my dad. We are very close, and his influence in my life has always been abundantly positive. True to form, his advice was clear, powerful, and true. He told me that eventually I was going to have to **spend money to make money**. In other words, I was going to have to invest in myself and my business in order for it to grow. Otherwise, it would stagnate and die.

Though the advice was excellent, for someone who does NOT like to spend money, this was really hard to hear. I started my cash practice for under $1000 overhead, and $500 of that was given to a lawyer to expedite my LLC so that I could see my first patient as soon as possible, legally (I told you, I'm not a rule breaker!). So, the idea of spending money to learn how to run a business, especially when I was on bedrest and not making any money, was hard to swallow. I wasn't even sure how I could afford to send my daughter to daycare (because I couldn't watch my own child while on bedrest), and I definitely had no idea how I was going to pay to learn from a business expert. Nevertheless, my dad convinced me that if I was serious about my business, it was time to invest in learning from those who had gone before me.

At this point, I knew I needed an expert teacher who had been there before. I figured, if I had all this time on bedrest, why don't I make the most of it and find someone who can teach me everything he or she knows. I needed to **learn absolutely everything** I could to fix my website and generate patients on my own, so that eventually, I would have a business to come back to once my son was born.

THAT BRITISH GUY

If you're going to do something, it's worth doing really well! With that in mind, I was dead set on putting my best foot forward as I grew my own practice. In addition to spending every waking moment consuming relevant reading materials, I was also binge-listening to every podcast about cash physical therapy. As I was starting on my journey, and while enthralled by Jarod Carter's podcast, *The Cash-Based Practice Podcast*, I stumbled on an interview with a British guy named Paul Gough. He made such an impression that I remember thinking, "if I ever get serious about my business, I'm going to learn from that guy."

Well, now I was serious, and it didn't take long for me to get hold of him. I emailed him, told him my situation, and then enrolled in his *Accelerator* course... I have never looked back since.

The owner of *Paul Gough Media* and *Paul Gough Physio Rooms* in Hartlepool, England, came to be one of the most amazing mentors in my professional career. I knew instantly that he would help me, and boy has he done that! Under his tutelage, I have grown not one, but *two* profitable physical therapy businesses.

MY EYES WERE OPENED

On my journey I have come to learn that everyone has a turning point, one at which he or she has a unique realization. Taking *Accelerator* was that turning point for me. I devoured the material while I was unable to work, spending all day (and night) implementing everything Paul taught me about marketing, communicating with patients, and follow-up systems. He helped me scrutinize my business and look at it in a way that I'd never thought of before.

Every single module of *Accelerator* was like opening a surprise Christmas gift.... and then I got to module 5... websites. Paul had me inspect my business from the standpoint of my website. Why was I getting ZERO enquiries? And on top of that, what do people do when they're considering doing business with me? They turn to my website, of course.

And that's the moment I realized that I was not leveraging one of the most powerful marketing tools in my business, one that could work for me 24/7, *even* while I was on bedrest. **My website had generated ZERO patients in the last year and a half.** Re-read that last sentence.

My website had generated ZERO patients in the last year and a half.

Everything stopped in that moment; how could I have gotten this so monumentally wrong? What was happening? Something had to be done, and it needed to be done immediately.

I knew that I would have to restart my little physical therapy business after the baby was born, and fixing my website – making it run and bring in patients – was the best way I could jump start the process. My mind was made up. I had no income to speak of, my family needed me, and I needed to find out how to rectify the mess of a website I had.

THE REBUILDING PROCESS

How did I transform my website into a patient-generating machine? I wasn't a web developer or trained in anything tech-savvy, so I turned to *Google*. But the craziest thing is, although I spent hours and hours trying to find someone who rebuilt their website from scratch, at home, by themselves, AND who had seen dramatic results, no one was to be found!

There was absolutely no one who had done what I wanted to do, that is, make their own website with "Paul-Style" physical therapy marketing. I looked everywhere; I was completely out of my depth and entirely alone in the process.

At that point, I had two options: *pay someone to help me* or *do it myself.* Because I was already on bedrest and unable to pursue my clinical practice, I really felt tight on cash. I had already spent money I didn't have on *Accelerator* and wasn't sure how or when I would be able to go back to work; I wasn't even sure I could afford daycare for both my children so that I could go back to work! My only other remaining option was to do it on my own – and that would take a lot of time and effort... and I mean A LOT.

Thankfully, my bedrest gave me an asset that most business owners don't have: it gave me **TIME**. Time is definitely not a commodity that everyone has – but, I had lots of it, and I was going to use it to my advantage.

The first thing that had to go was my beautiful picture of the woman and the sunset. I had to do away with the frills in order to get down to the *nitty gritty* of it all. And yet, I can't deny that I cringed a little bit as I deconstructed my "beautiful and professional" website. I had spent weeks building my company's online presence only to see it completely and utterly fail. Through gritted teeth I acknowledged that, in order for my business to survive, my website had to be revamped from the bottom up.

With that first hurdle was overcome, I spent hours and hours studying what it means to build a patient-generating website and how to do all of the technology aspects by myself. I did all this without understanding coding or having learned how to code like a web developer. Though by no means easy, I've always enjoyed a good challenge, and it was a fulfilling and satisfying task; I was pushing myself and growing in a way that I had never known, and I was excited to see the fruits of my labor benefiting my business.

I implemented the new knowledge, built my new website, said a prayer, and put it online for the world to take notice of shortly after my son, Jackson, was born. I was nervous, of course, but I realized I couldn't go back to the outdated, unsuccessful website I had been using – this was it, it had to work. People had to notice... and boy, did they notice.

THE LAUNCH

Shortly after the launch of my website, people suddenly started inquiring in droves. In the first year I had over 100 new patient leads *without* any paid advertising (of course, the number was higher when paid advertising was added!). People started filling out the forms. They downloaded the freebies. They were calling my office and saying "I knew you were right for me because of your website." They were SEEING my business and how I could solve their problems. And all I could think at the time was... "this is crazy."

Quite apart from the phenomenal awareness my website created for my small business, it was the profound reaction I got from the visitors (who later became patients) that really got me. People kept coming up to me or writing to me, saying things like, "Your website spoke to me. I knew you were the right person to help me." For someone who was new to the world of website design, who was really a novice learning how to market her physical therapy practice, this outcome was staggering.

PT WEBSITE SUCCESS

There I was, having come though some of the toughest things I have ever had to experience in my life, and I was standing tall. For the first time I honestly felt as though my practice, my business, my finances, and my *dream* was going to make it! I had more new patient inquiries than ever before and many of them were converting to new patients! I was ready to keep running full steam ahead.

Importantly, the response to my website really showed me that my marketing education to date was working. I could see it in action right there on my website. It was as though a lightbulb went off in my head: I knew how to do this. I, as a physical therapist with no technological background, could be a web designer. I learned the skills, had the passion, and implemented what needed to be done – I did it.

I was so overwhelmed by the positive response to my website and what it meant for my clinic, that I hadn't even begun to realize what it meant for me, personally. Little did I grasp the overall power of my website, and less still did I know how my personal growth in website design would lead me down an altogether different career path.

As my website was growing, my cash practice was doing the same. It was always my goal to grow my cash practice successfully enough to hit the ground running straight after my pregnancy. While this did indeed happen, another interesting thing also occurred. I started getting calls, not about my clinic, but from other physical therapists asking questions about how to build a website!

I had at this point been part of the *Accelerator* course, and, because of my success with the program, I furthered my involvement by joining Paul's *Mastermind* the *4% Club*™. Throughout my own journey, as well as throughout *Accelerator*, I had already started making contacts and life-long friends, many of whom were now asking me for website advice!

It soon became clear that many of the people I'd met along the way were very interested in building or transforming their websites, and more amazing still, they seemed to regard me as someone who knew how. I needed to note this very important shift.

28

One thing I learned from Paul early on in my career is that, as a PT, you should listen to your patients and the questions they are asking, because that's what you should blog about and use as your marketing material. Don't complicate content such as your blogs, just answer the questions people are asking you. And suddenly it dawned on me: so many people are asking me about building websites... why am I not answering their questions?!

PT WEBSITE SECRETS™ IS BORN

It was then that my life changed in a way I could not have foreseen two years prior. It became so abundantly clear that THIS physical therapy website building, designing, and education, was the way in which I could **help** people most. I knew immediately that this is how I needed to enrich the lives of the people I met along the way.

The most amazing thing about this journey is that, as a physical therapist, I could only help so many patients each week - my time was limited. But I could help other PT's reach more people with their online presence!

I knew that there are many amazingly skilled physical therapists who can help free people from their chronic back pain, women's health issues, or help their patients achieve the personal record they're looking for in the *Crossfit* box, the only problem is that their websites weren't attracting those patients; people kept suffering unnecessarily. What I then realized was that by helping other physical therapy business owners get the right patients off of the internet and into their clinics, then our impact can be greater together.

In October 2017, I made my first website sale and in November 2017 I first launched my signature online course, *The Workshop*. *PT Website Secrets™* was born. Since then, I've helped over 100 physical therapists build or revamp their clinic's websites, sites which have led to the conversions of thousands of patients across the country who wouldn't have ended up in a physical therapist's office otherwise.

It brings me such joy to see the significant improvement in these physical therapy businesses, not only in their finances, but in the personal lives of the PT owner's themselves!

One thing I've enjoyed most about this journey is seeing the staggering results my clients have experienced in their own businesses, and even more than that, how these changes have positively affected their lives. For example, the dearly loved Kris Winders, founder of *BBN Physical Therapy*, is now making an extra $3,000 a month, without any additional marketing, from ONE of the many changes we made to his clinic's website.

Paul Jones, *Jones Physical Therapy*, is another one of those success stories. After having a brochure-style website transformed with the *PT Website Secrets™ System*, he went from zero online leads in YEARS to **10 new patient appointments in 12 days after launching his new site** - a 900% return on his investment in less than two weeks! To this day he continues to get at least 5 new patients from his website each week.

This can be you, too. I want you to have the same success, and that is why, in this powerful book, I'm going to share with you my *PT Website Secrets™ System*. I want to show you how to build a successful, sustainable, BUSINESS BUILDING website you can be proud of.

YOUR STORY

I didn't write this book to try to make you happy, content, or feel good about what you have on your PT website. I've written this book to challenge you to take a hard look at your physical therapy website and ask yourself, *"what if I could make this better?"*

My challenge to you is this: instead of thinking "this could never work for me," or "I don't know how I could ever do this," or "this makes me really uncomfortable," I want you to think, "what if this could work for me? What would that do for my life and my business?" I want you to make the change that will CHANGE YOUR LIFE.

If you're serious about taking the steps needed to make your website WORK for you, if you're ready to see your business transform and your website become the BEST employee you have, and if you're ready to sleep well at night KNOWING that you will have patients the next day, then let's get started. The *PT Website Secret System* is for YOU!

Are you ready to learn the *PT Website Secrets™ System*? Let's go!

3

THE POWER
OF THE RIGHT WEBSITE

Now that you know my story, and you're beginning to understand how important having a working, profitable website is, it's time get down to the nitty gritty of the *PTWS System*. But, before we do, we need to address an incredibly important question:

WHY DO YOU HAVE A WEBSITE FOR YOUR PHYSICAL THERAPY CLINIC?

This may seem like a silly question, initially, but think carefully about it... what is your motivation for having a website for your physical therapy clinic? Though it seems self-explanatory, most physical therapist really don't seem to have a clear answer. Do you?

So many of the people who contact me about building their websites are surprised by my approach. First off, I make a point of getting to know everything there is to know about their businesses – from origins, to specializations, to owners' motivations. Knowing everything there is to know is absolutely vital in conceptualizing a website. Why? Because, if I don't know what your business is, where you want it to go, and who specifically you serve, then I can't give you any advice on how to improve your website in order to get you the results you desire.

You're probably thinking, "why is this information so crucial to your website's development?" Good question. Aren't we just trying to put our business online so that people can find us and call us? Though this might seem like the logical reason for having a website, this type of thinking exposes a real problem in the industry: *physical therapy clinic owners don't understand why they should have a website in the first place.*

WHY DO YOU HAVE A WEBSITE?

When you first started your business, you probably felt like you needed to have a website *before* you started seeing patients. You're not alone! Most PT owners feel the same.

I say "most" because there are, of course, PT owners who are the exception, such as people who started prior to the Internet boom. I have one client who has had a cash PT practice for over 25 years! Yet, in the world of today – one that is run by technology and a startling need for speed – if you're not on the internet, then people assume you're not legitimate (or maybe worse, that you're lazy). That's how people think.

Knowing this, most PT owners find themselves in a mad rush to get a website. Why? Well, apart from societal dictates, I've found that there are three reasons people *build* a website or *pay* someone else to do it:

1. To prove he or she has a real business.
2. So people can find him or her and call.
3. Because he or she thought a website was a necessity.

All of these reasons give a very limited view on the power of a website. It's almost like saying, "I love my car because I can listen to the radio in it," but you never actually take your car out of the driveway or use it to drive anywhere. So many websites are like new, *stationary* cars, lined up with their radios blaring from the windows. Most people are simply not utilizing the full capacity of their websites. Their websites aren't doing the ONE THING they're meant to do – grow their businesses!

NOW IS THE TIME TO BE ONLINE

As I'm writing this chapter, I'm sitting at *Panera* and taking in my surroundings. A man in a green hat just walked by on my left. He's heading to another store and he's looking down, staring intently at his phone, likely browsing the internet. Two other businessmen are sipping on coffees, laptops out, having a serious discussion. Suddenly, one of them is interrupted by a random alert on his phone, probably an email. On my right side, two women are laughing while they watch a video on their phones. Everyone, everywhere, is attached to the internet. We take it with us when we go shopping, go to meetings, attend our kids' sporting events – there is literally NO escape.

What a time to be a business owner! There has never been a better time to grow your business with the help of your website. On average, Americans spend more than 20 hours a week online, and almost every one of those people access the internet through their smartphones. Your business is waiting to be accessed right at the fingertips of every passerby! It is almost too easy to get in front of people today – the internet has made accessibility so common that grabbing the attention of potential patients is not only possible, it's GUARANTEED with the right website. What do I mean by the right website? Well, the secret is to know and understand *what people actually want to do on the internet.*

THE 3 MAIN REASONS PEOPLE
USE THE INTERNET

As millions of people handle their smartphones, surf the internet in crowded coffee shops, or sit down to the desktops in their offices, we have to ask ourselves – what is it that they're doing on the internet? Once we know that, we're one step closer to understanding what will make your website work. Here are the three main reasons people use the Internet:

#1: To be Entertained and to Kill Time

If I had a penny for every time I've heard my four-year-old daughter say "I'm BORED!" well, I would be a seriously rich woman. And when she's bored, her instinct is to reach for the *iPad*. Admittedly, this bugs me a lot, but then I realize that I'm just as guilty. In today's world, boredom is the realm of the Internet. Let's face it, when we're watching television and a commercial comes on, or we're stuck in a traffic jam, or we're struggling to sleep, the majority of us reach for our smartphones or tablets. It's instinctual in the 21st century. For right or for wrong, most people around the world access the internet in moments of boredom. And why is this? Because we want to be **entertained**!

#2: To Avoid Doing Something

A close cousin of boredom is procrastination. How often have you found yourself reading the news headlines for the seventh time in an hour to avoid doing the dishes? Or, when you have to wash the car or mow the lawn, how often have you been caught up in a website that engrosses you *just then*? Like most other people, you probably find yourself endlessly browsing the internet when you know you should be doing something else. Maybe you're dreading calling back a prospective patient and having the "do you take my insurance" conversation. So, what do you do? You reach for the smartphone instead.

Your brain is wired to avoid discomfort, and the internet is the easiest and most entertaining way to avoid doing the things you don't want to do.

Let's take this notion back to your website and your potential patients for a moment. Think about it: so many of the people you can help, the people with back pain, knee pain, and/or neck pain are trying to avoid thinking about their problems by being on the internet. Shouldn't your website be aware of this? And shouldn't your website be acutely focused on the next reason...

#3: To Find Solutions to Their Problems

Here's an example of how this has played out in my personal life. In early 2018, I find myself crawling into bed at 10:00 PM. My kids are FINALLY asleep, this after my daughter performed her excellent stalling tactics to keep me in the room as long as possible. My son, on the other hand, is sick again. It never seems to end. It seems to be one illness after another, all of which are spiking serious fevers in the wake of common colds. He doesn't seem to be getting better without multiple antibiotic regimes.

Our pediatrician has been running tests; she suspects that it's more than "daycare-itis" and that he's not sick only because of his constant exposure to other kids. Her latest attempt is to test him for IG deficiencies. Until now, I haven't had time to sit down and read about this possible diagnosis, so as I prepare for bed I pull out my phone and start *Google*-ing.

The websites that draw my attention are super informative, having lots of free information about IG testing and immunodeficiency. Some even have free information that I can download or have sent to my email. I opt-in to a few resources so that I can research this problem in-depth tomorrow, when I'm less tired.

I'm sure you can think of a time and situation where you have done something very similar. What problem or question have you had that prompted you to whip out your phone and search for the solution on the Internet?

You're not alone.

Decades ago the library and encyclopedia were the closest we could get to accessing information on such a broad scale, but now there are so many resources at our fingertips. Your potential patients are on the internet looking for solutions to their problems even as I'm writing this. They want to know why their backs are aching after 18 holes of golf or whether there is an easier way to get off the floor after they play with their grandchildren. The Internet is where they go looking for these solutions. Shouldn't you be supplying them with the answers?

. . .

Looking at these 3 dominant reasons for internet use, it's no wonder that I'm driven crazy by the fact that 99% of physical therapy websites have been built WITHOUT considering HOW people actually use the internet. When was the last time you saw a physical therapy clinic's website that was entertaining or interesting enough to access when you're bored or procrastinating?

Even worse, how many PT websites actually provide solutions to problems, actually explaining what's going on in a way that a patient can understand, instead of with technical and medical terms?

Most companies, especially physical therapy businesses, don't actually design their websites for functionality. PT websites are often not the type of place bored, procrastinating, or desperate people would want to visit and/or stay on for a duration of time. And that's precisely why so many PT clinics have a hard time getting new patients from the Internet.

WE USE THE INTERNET FOR US

The common denominator is that we use the internet for ourselves. No matter whether we are trying to burn time, be entertained, or solve problems, the goal is to accomplish something for ourselves, personally. Seldom do we use the Internet to solve problems for relatives who live hours away, or for strangers we hardly know. Instead, we access the Internet to better our OWN lives or the lives of those closest to us.

As humans, we're wired to survive. Whether you consciously think about it or not, all the decisions you make in a day are always held up to the benchmark, "is this going to help me survive?" It's our primal instinct, and it's a good one if we want the human race to continue.

When you or I use the internet, we're subconsciously filtering all the information through that ideal survival standard. It makes sense that our Internet usage reflects our instinctive need to better our own lives in the hope of survival. We may have our moments of empathy or altruism, but really we use the internet for ourselves and for our own benefit. And that's why most physical therapy websites don't get our attention. **They don't talk to us in a way that makes us feel their content is necessary for our survival.**

I can think, for example, about someone in my family who has nagging back pain which comes and goes depending on how many times she lifts her grandchildren. She really needs to do something about her back pain before it becomes a debilitating issue, but she doesn't realize the full impact that physical therapy would have on her problem. Instead, back pain keeps her awake at night; she wonders if she's doomed to suffer through this for the rest of her life.

Why doesn't she understand what a beneficial role physical therapy will play in the health of her back? Well, if she's on the internet looking at ways to ease her back pain, and she comes across one (or a combination of) the traditional physical therapy websites out there, do you think she's going to clear her busy schedule and book an appointment? Nope.

Let's say she finds a website whose main message is that their physical therapy clinic is amazing and that she'll be treated 1-on-1 by a professional, friendly, caring, qualified physical therapist who, by the way, has 20 years of experience. Is that message convincing her in any way, shape, or form that something can actually be done to help her with her back pain? Nope.

Or how about if she comes across a website that talks about how back pain can be cured with manual therapy, therapeutic exercise, and a customized plan of care? Will that entice her to take time out of her busy day, spend money, and do something about her back pain? Nope.

And what about if she comes across a website that promises they can fix any problem - orthopedic, neurological, or pediatric? Well, we'll see the same result. She won't be impressed by the fact that someone can treat every diagnosis possible. She needs a back pain specialist. Yet instead of that, she'll be overwhelmed; she'll not take action, thereby letting her back pain continue for even longer.

ONCE AGAIN, WHY DO YOU HAVE A WEBSITE?

So I'll ask you again – why do you, as a PT owner, have a website? As I hinted at the beginning of this chapter, the biggest problem with most PT websites is that the PT owner doesn't consider why it is that he or she has a website to begin with.

Let's start here: I'm confident that universally all PT business owners want more patients. We want our websites to do more than prove we exist, we want them to go beyond being a beacon of hope for the phone line to lean on. We want our websites to help us grow our businesses!

Many of us are knocked down by the poor performance of our website. We believe our standards were too high and so we lower our expectations to offset or ignore the problem all together, to cover our disappointment. We've either spent a lot of money or time on our website, and therefore we try to make ourselves feel better by believing that other people must not be getting new patients from online either, so it must be okay.

This attitude is selling yourself and your business short. In fact, this type of thinking leads you to not realizing the power your website has to get your new patients. In truth, your website is so powerful that it should be the foundation of your entire business! You just need to understand why you need one.

WHY YOUR WEBSITE IS YOUR BUSINESS'S FOUNDATION

Your website lays the foundation for a strong, powerful, profitable, functional business. Let's think about this for a second. What's the first thing do you do when your best friend tells you about an amazing new restaurant? Look it up online, of course. What did I do when my aunt suggested we take my kids to the new trampoline park in her town? I looked it up online to see if it would be a good fit for my kids!

It used to be that the opinion of your friend or family member was enough to get you to take action without question. If your mom said to go see this dentist, you did, because of course your mom knows best. But that's no longer the case. We all want to do our own research; we want to read the reviews of others and to see for ourselves whether or not we think the business in question is a good fit for us. We want to be the judge. And how do we do that? We visit a business's website.

Your website is the foundational structure which draws in and secures potential patients. It needs to be good enough to fulfill this function.

And yet, astonishingly, many people think they can overcome an average website with really good marketing. I want to show you why this is not the case.

IF DISNEY WERE A DUMP...

We all know that *Disney World* is far from being "a dump," but bear with me for one minute. Imagine seeing all the signs and advertisements for *Disney* and thinking how amazing this place must be. *Disney's* marketing almost makes you believe that magic and fantasy could be real. Your kids are excited, and you even find yourself anticipating an amazing vacation with your family.

But what would happen if, after seeing all the amazing advertisements, you showed up and found *Disney* to be a complete dump? Imagine if *Disney* was run-down with weeds growing everywhere, with half of the rides closed for maintenance, and with only one man taking tickets so you have to wait outside for hours just to get in? Would you recommend *Disney* to your friends and family? Would you tell them to go? ABSOLUTELY NOT.

As Simon Godding (of *Paul Gough Media*), marketing expert for top PTs across the US, explains:

> "Marketing BEFORE your PT website is done right
> is like inviting people to the opening night of your
> new restaurant, but giving the chef the night off."

In other words, you're losing a lot of clients by not being ready for their visits to your website. Remember, the car analogy? Your potential patients see your website, but all they can hear is blaring music and very little of ANYTHING that they actually want or need. The car, aka you website, hasn't even moved out of the driveway.

If you have an awesome service but a crappy website, your marketing efforts will be less effective because your website undermines all the good work you've put in. Your potential clients think they're getting the magic akin to *Disney*, yet are disappointed when they actually look you up online. Your potential for converting paying customers drops significantly at the hands of a dysfunctional website.

How does this apply to your own practice right now? Well, if you're out talking to yoga and fitness studios, hosting workshops, going to community events, handing out business cards, or even joining networking groups, then you're marketing. If you're posting on social media, sending emails, or running *Facebook* and *Google* ads, then you're definitely marketing. And assuming you're marketing effectively, what do your potential patients do after their interest in your business has been peaked? They go to the website to get more information.

It's the whole *Disney* dilemma again. Even when your marketing is amazing, people are instinctively going to go look at your website before they decide to do business with you. And if your website is only pretty and professional, then you aren't giving your potential patients the information they want, and you're not going to convert to paying patients. Those patients will not be clicking your "book now" button... they're not ready or comfortable yet to take that leap.

YOUR WEBSITE IS NOT FOR BOOKING NEW PATIENTS

I'm going to let you in on a secret that is going to change your entire perspective of your website. The biggest mistake you can make is to assume your website's purpose is to book new patients. It's not. In fact, **85% of people are NOT ready to book or call you after first seeing your website** (in fact, we're going to talk a lot more about this in Chapter 9).

Yes, it's true. When I first started my cash practice, I didn't know this fact. I definitely thought that my website should be creating an environment that would, firstly, encourage patients to call me *immediately*, or secondly, book online without having a conversation with me.

And that is why I made the mistake of designing my first website in the way I described in Chapter 1. I made sure to explain all about my practice, how it was different, why it was cash-based, and how much treatment would cost. Why? I believed those words would convince people to do business with me. In other words, I was trying to avoid having the tough conversations on the phone... like "do you take my insurance?"

So, with all that information on my website, I thought I would have it easy. Patients would book on my website and be willing to pay cash for my services...sounds like a dream, right? Yes, but that's because *it is a dream*. I've tried it and *that* patient ended up not understanding anything about my clinic and turning out to be a bad fit overall.

The bottom line is you're not going to be able to grow and scale a business by booking new cash paying patients straight from your website. It's almost like asking someone to marry you without ever having met in person. That's messy – really messy.

Please note – I'm not talking about past patients in this section. I'm referring to new patients who find you online and know nothing about your business.

Most physical therapy websites make the mistake of giving the same ultimatum. You can either book or call now, or hit the back button. And guess what? When given an ultimatum, almost all website visitors hit the back button.

And that is why, if you don't have your website nailed, it doesn't matter how much successful marketing you are doing. No matter how many workshops you put on, yoga studios you visit, or doctors' lunches you provide, people will go look you up online afterwards before they make a decision to commit to come and see you. And, if your website is not right, those patients aren't going to do business with you, and you're going to get stuck – you'll be unable to grow your company any further.

You may hit that roadblock at three to five patients a week (like me), or maybe it will happen later when you're at ten to fifteen patients – or it might even happen when you're looking to hire your next therapist. It's really scary to be stuck wondering when the next new patient is going to come and not knowing where he or she is going to come *from*. And that's why you need to get your website transformed, right now.

IT'S TIME TO LOOK IN THE MIRROR

Now it's time to ask yourself the hard question. It's time to put aside your pride. Put aside your need for validation that all the money you spent on physical therapy school was worth it, and honestly ask yourself, "why do you really have a website?"

Do you want to have a website that displays all your accolades, accomplishments, skills, and training?

Or do you want to have a website that is made for your potential patients – one that is functional and informative? Do you want a website that is made for growing the type of business that will give you the lifestyle and career you desire?

Are you willing to give up your pretty professional website? That is, are you willing to let go of the website that makes *you* look amazing, but really does nothing to get new *patients* in the door or increase the number of times the phone rings?

Are you willing to stop talking about your specialized treatment techniques, and instead talk about your patients and their deepest desires and fears?

I've met a lot of people who aren't ready to tackle these questions. They're so invested in their current websites, whether it's how it looks, what it says, or the professional photo shoot they paid for, that they can't give it up. They can't stand the idea of starting over. If that's you, *then you're not ready for this book.* If you're not willing to let the "pretty" go in order to reach the people I KNOW you can help, right now, then these pages aren't for you.

But if you are ready to change your business, change your website, and change your life, then I'm excited to have you join me on this journey to transform your physical therapy website into a patient-generating machine. The time is now – your website can be your greatest employee and your greatest asset. Ask yourself the difficult questions, make the commitment, and let's overhaul your online presence once and for all. I know you can do it!

I hope you're excited, because I sure am! Let's dive into the *PT Website Secrets™ System.*

4

THE PT WEBSITE SECRETS™ SYSTEM

In the previous chapters we touched on the benefits and reasoning behind having a lead-generating website, so it's now time to turn our attention to getting your own website up and running! We'll be looking at the *PT Website Secrets™ System* in this chapter, and you'll get a taste of what lies in store for your website and business.

Before we get to the nitty gritty of the system, I want you to be aware of something. There are two types of physical therapy practices: those who rely on referrals for new patients and those who don't.

Those who rely on referrals, whether from physicians or other healthcare professionals, gyms, yoga or Pilates studios, have to hustle day in and day out to maintain good relationships with their patient referral sources. It's vital that these practices stay on the minds of the people who refer to their PT businesses. If their referral sources forget about their clinics, or if they no longer feel validated or supported by the PT clinics in question, the PT practices will see referrals drop; their businesses will suffer. It's a tough cycle to be stuck in.

These types of physical therapy businesses, which rely on patient referrals, include not only the big hospital systems which get their new patients from in-house physicians but also the new cash practice gyms which, for example, get 75% of their patients from gym memberships.

I'm going to be brutally honest. This book is not for the type of business that's *content* to rely on referrals for new patients. Why? Because these types of clinics risk their business's stability by relying on temperamental, fickle referral sources. We won't worry about them in this book... unless they're willing and eager to <u>decrease this dependency</u> and learn ways to generate business through website marketing – a platform so much more reliable, profitable, and functional than old-school hustling.

This book is for the PT business owner who has a FIRE in himself or herself for breaking free of referral dependence. And if you're already there, great! These pages are specifically written for owners who are EXCITED about being able to create dependable, predictable, profitable leads via websites that work! Whether you're starting on your journey or you are halfway up the mountain, these chapters are here to help you reach your goal of a successful, profitable, reliable business through the use of your website. Let me show you how it's done.

WHO OWNS YOUR BUSINESS?

Whoever owns your traffic, owns your business.

Think about this statement for a moment. What does it mean? Let me ask you two questions:

- Are you reliant on word-of-mouth referrals? Are you constantly asking patients to tell their friends and family about you? Is that where the bulk of your new patients come from? If so, then your patients own your business.
- Do you get your new patients through referrals from other providers? Examples of these types of *providers* are physicians, fitness studios, gyms, massage therapists, chiropractors, or any other person/people providing a service. If so, then these professionals own your business.

If you're answering yes to the above two questions, you DO NOT own your traffic. And if you do not have control over how your new patients walk through you clinic's doors, you definitely are not in control of your own business. Those you rely on to refer your services are the real owners. They own your business, not you. Remember, **those who own the traffic, own the business!**

The number one reason new PT clinics fail is because the PT owners don't actually own the business. These PT clinics are at the mercy of the real owners, those who refer, who are unpredictable, inconstant, and unreliable. Being at the mercy of others is like hoping it will rain during a drought – it might, but you can't rely on it. You cannot predict referrals in this situation, and your business is in a constant state of flux. This is NOT a way to be profitable and grow a business.

We need to get your business to a place where the answer to both the questions above is an emphatic, "NO!" True independence and profitability comes from being able to generate, predict, and rely on profitable, consistent leads. When YOU are generating leads and converting patients with a direct-to-patient marketing strategy, that's when you know that YOU, and you alone, own your business.

And how do you do this? Yes, you guessed it – your website. More than almost anything else, your website will determine whether YOU, or those who refer to you, own your business. It's *that* important.

WHERE ARE YOU ON THE JOURNEY TO OWNING YOUR BUSINESS?

Now, I realize that many of you reading this book are at different stages in your journey to independence from referrals. Remember that what matters is not where you are, it's where you're going. No matter where you find yourself in your move towards truly owning your business, you're making that decision and it will change your life for the better.

Take a look at the picture below. I call this the *Ownership Mountain*, and in it I've illustrated the different stages that PT owners find themselves in on their respective journeys to start, grow, and sustain a profitable business.

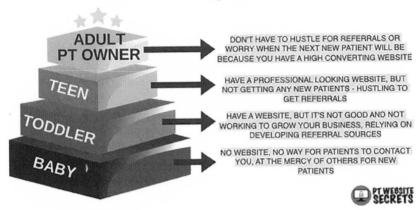

The Ownership Mountain

ADULT PT OWNER → DON'T HAVE TO HUSTLE FOR REFERRALS OR WORRY WHEN THE NEXT NEW PATIENT WILL BE BECAUSE YOU HAVE A HIGH CONVERTING WEBSITE

TEEN → HAVE A PROFESSIONAL LOOKING WEBSITE, BUT NOT GETTING ANY NEW PATIENTS - HUSTLING TO GET REFERRALS

TODDLER → HAVE A WEBSITE, BUT IT'S NOT GOOD AND NOT WORKING TO GROW YOUR BUSINESS, RELYING ON DEVELOPING REFERRAL SOURCES

BABY → NO WEBSITE, NO WAY FOR PATIENTS TO CONTACT YOU, AT THE MERCY OF OTHERS FOR NEW PATIENTS

PT WEBSITE SECRETS

Baby - Ownership babies don't even have a website. They have no way for their patients or prospective patients to contact them when they are looked up online. Babies are at the complete mercy of others for new patient referrals. And, like infants who are at the mercy of their parents for food, safety, and mobility, these ownership babies are completely dependent on third party referrals.

Toddler - Toddlers have graduated up the ownership mountain and they have websites. The only problem is, they're not very good. These websites aren't doing anything to help grow their businesses, so ownership toddlers are still reliant on outside referral sources to survive. Like real life toddlers, they may be able to get out and walk a little, but a trip to the zoo is going to require their parents to push them around in strollers.

Teen – Ownership teenagers have professional-looking websites, but, like all actual teens, they're obsessed with their looks! At this point in the journey, owners incorrectly think that "being good-looking" is what will bring them success in life. Their clinics' websites still aren't working, though, so the teenagers are hustling hard, and experiencing major stress, to find patients in order to grow their businesses.

Adult Business Owners - Adult business owners have learned the secrets. They don't have to hustle anymore, and can get home for dinner by 5 PM, thereby spending time with their young kids if they desire. They don't worry about when or where the next new patient will come from, because they have their website set-up to predictably bring in new patients. They have a high-converting website that gets traffic and turns website visits into new patient inquiries.

Take a close look at the *Ownership Mountain*. These 4 stages are fundamental in understanding where you are right now, and where you are going. If you're a baby, don't worry – by reading this book you have taken a giant developmental leap on your way to adulthood and true ownership. Think about what you want from this process, where you want to be, and your commitment to achieving your goals. These pages will help you get there.

The purpose of this book, therefore, is to show you the roadmap for going from toddler or teen to adult physical therapy business owner. The steps you need to take are within reach, and I encourage you to commit wholeheartedly to the process.

I know you're dying to know the answer to the million dollar question:

> *How do you get a website that consistently brings in new patient leads so that you aren't reliant on other people for your business to grow... so that you OWN your business?*

Great question, and it's precisely this type of enquiry that drove me to create the *PT Website Secrets™ System*. In the second half of this chapter I'm going to give you an overview of the process, while the remainder of the book dives into the system's steps in greater detail.

PT WEBSITE SECRETS™ *SYSTEM*: THREE PARTS

What's the first thing we do when we think about building a website? We reach for the computer, right? Wrong. I'm a firm believer in building your website completely OFFLINE before ever opening up an internet browser to start work on the actual website. The website platform you use, or how fancy your website looks, is not going to determine whether or not your website will help to grow your business and bring in more new patients.

With this in mind, I'm going to explain the process I take with my private clients to build their patient-generating profitable websites. You'll notice that first part, which is what I spend the most time on (and which is the focus of this book), is not designing the website. That doesn't come till the second part of the process. The key to this entire process is part #1.

Here are the three processes I use in the *PT Website Secrets*™ *System*:

1. **Strategize**
2. **Design**
3. **Optimize**

The purpose of this book is to cover the majority of the strategize portion, or process #1, of this system, as it would be impossible for me to completely map out the design and optimization process in one book! Yet, remember, step number one – strategize – is the most important component of the entire system.

The design portion, process #2, of the *PT Website Secrets*™ *System* is the actual building of the website online. This is where we take all of the puzzle pieces we strategized in process #1 and actually put the puzzle together! These steps are discussed in step-by-step detail in a lesson in of my signature online course, *The Workshop.*

Process #3, Optimize, is the most important step for your long-term success. You must treat your website like any other employee, and be constantly monitoring its progress and teaching it new skills. I work closely with PT business owners both in group and 1-on-1 settings to continually improve and adapt their websites so that they are up-to-date with the latest successful online marketing strategies. I will give you an overview of the optimization process in Chapter 10.

To complete part #1, strategize, we use the 6 *PT Website Secrets*™ Questions and Principles to guide us. Take a look.

THE 6 FUNDAMENTALS OF THE PT WEBSITE SECRETS™ SYSTEM

You'll see that the 6 fundamentals of the *PT Website Secrets*™ *System* are structured as questions and, in addition, I have accompanied each question with an overarching principle. Why? Because I want you to remember that every part of this process is an opportunity for self-reflection. In other words, I want you to always consider the position of your website against that of your ideal patient – if you're answering the questions for YOUR PATIENTS, then you're on the right track. And if you have a principle to guide you to the answer, even better. Here are your 6 overarching questions and principles:

Question #1: "What are you selling?"

This is an essential step in strategizing your website. What are you selling? Don't be afraid that I used the word selling to talk about physical therapy. Let's get one thing straight: we are *selling* physical therapy, like your mom was selling an 8 PM bedtime when you were a kid. We *sell* people products, ideas, or even simpler things like going to see a new movie with us. So, why don't we have the selling mentality in physical therapy?

The problem is that most physical therapists think they are selling ONLY physical therapy. When you sell physical therapy alone, you become like every other physical therapy clinic in town. And that means you can be compared and, even worse, price shopped! Your competition is literally every other physical therapy clinic in town, and that's an awful place to be. So, I'm going to ask you again – what are you selling?

The first thing I determine with all my private clients is what they are selling. In other words, what makes them unique? The biggest problem is that many of them don't know. They think that, because they focus on hands-on therapy, or work 1-on-1 with clients, they are different. They're not, and the key to success is finding precisely what it is that makes them stand out – makes them different and WORTH paying for. Finding the answer to the question, "what am I selling?" is the foundation of building your website.

As we delve deeper into the *PT Website Secrets*™ *System*, I'll show you how to figure out what you are selling in your PT business.

Principle #1: *Don't Sell Physical Therapy. Sell Solutions to Problems*

Question #2: "Who are you selling to?"

Once you know *what* you are selling, you then need to figure out *who* you are selling your superior physical therapy services to. At a glance, it may seem obvious, right? You're selling to patients, aren't you? Yes and no. "Patients" is a very broad concept, and the belief that you are selling to ALL patients may, in fact, be limiting; it might even hold you back from great success.

Let me explain. No one wants to see the physical therapist who can fix everything. If you can fix everything then you're great at nothing. So, if your potential client visits your website only to see that you do not cater to him or her specifically, he or she will click the back button and *Google* a specialist instead.

Truly, "the riches are in the niches," and if you try to sell to *everyone* you will end up selling to *no one*. People these days want specialists. They want to do business with people who have experience with their specific type of problem.

For this reason, you don't want to please everyone. The best websites are the ones that rule out a portion of their visitors! When you're building your website, you have to make every decision based on the group of people you want to serve.

So, the question, "who are you selling to?" is vitally important in creating a successful, informative, and profitable website.

Principle #2: *If You Try To Please Everyone, You Attract No One*

Question #3: How will you get their attention?

After identifying what you are selling and who you are selling to, the next thing to consider is how you will get their attention.

I want you to think about something. How many advertisements have you seen today? How many have you heard? You may even have smelled one! We are constantly and incessantly bombarded with messages, offers, and advertisements which are all aimed at getting us to take action. This is the overwhelming reality, and in the midst of all that chaos, our brains have learned to tune out the majority of what we hear.

So, I ask you this: what is going to make your offer stand out to the right people?

How are you going to avoid becoming part of the white noise created by the marketing industry?

In order to find the answer to this question, I've ensured that this step is all about figuring out what will engage YOUR audience and entice those people who are the best fit for your physical therapy business. Many businesses make the crucial mistake of skipping this step. They assume that their potential patients know that physical therapy can help. They even assume that patients actually understand what physical therapy is! Sadly, both these assumptions are very, very wrong.

With that in mind, what about your business is going to be *so* appealing that potential patients are willing to put down their phones, reorganize their schedules, and consider booking an appointment? Are they going to do this for something they only somewhat understand? No.

My calendar is sacred and usually not very flexible. Many other people feel the same way about their daily routines and commitments. You're going to have to have a super strong and clear message to appeal to your ideal patient group. You'll need to be very persuasive in order to convince them to commit to something like physical therapy, not least because it's a commitment which could very well take a significant amount of time to yield benefits.

Principle #3: *People Don't Pay Attention To (Or Buy) Things They Don't Understand*

Question #4: What will you offer?

As you've seen throughout the previous chapters, few patients are generally ready to take action immediately. We know from website research that about 15% of all visitors will be ready to take action and do something about their problem right now. Yet, the problem isn't so much the size of the percentage bracket, it's the fact that most patients who are ready don't actually want to "call now" or "book an appointment."

It's hard to blame them, really. We don't like picking up the phone either! I dread having to call a healthcare office to make any appointment. When was the last time you had a positive experience doing so? Calling a business, especially a healthcare business, is sometimes awkward or stressful, and often it's downright inconvenient.

In order to capture the 15% who are ready to fix their problems and consider physical therapy, we need to give them options. In this step, I'll show you how to give your website visitors options so as to eradicate the binary thinking of "call now" or "book an appointment." Remember, you're selling superior services – why not give your potential patients superior options that speak directly to their needs and desires? In other words, give yourself the best possible chance of netting in the entire 15% who are ready to make a commitment.

Principle #4: *People Won't Take Action Unless You Ask*

Question #5: What will you offer those who aren't ready yet?

Now that you know only 15% of potential patients are ready to contact you right now, what do you do about the remaining 85%? Surely we can't leave them to come around on their own? Of course not.

The growth and survival of your business will hinge on your ability to get the remaining 85% to become paying patients.

The challenge lies in the fact that these people are often skeptical, may have had a bad experience with a physical therapist in the past, or may not know enough to probe further, despite their interest in solving their problem.

So, what do you need to do? You have to "give before you get" with the 85% by giving them options as well, or else you'll lose them to other places like Dr. *Google, YouTube,* or your competitor down the street who, by the way, is willing to wait longer for them to become a patient.

In this step I show you how you can start relationships by offering other free information that potential patients can download by giving their contact details. Why? So that you can nurture trust through a real relationship with the 85% who aren't ready to do business, but who want more information. This is the *fortune* you will draw on and continue to nurture over the coming months... until they become patients.

Principle #5: *Revenue Results From Real Relationships*

Question #6: What's the end goal of your website?

How do you judge if your website is working? How do you judge if you're website is a success? I hear these questions all the time, and the answer is simple.

Your website has one sole purpose: to bring in new patient leads for your physical therapy business. Without being able to predictably generate leads on your own, you don't own your business and you won't be able to grow and scale in order to achieve the lifestyle of your dreams.

If your website isn't bringing in new patient leads, then your website isn't working and you're wasting valuable marketing resources online.

No website is ever perfect, including mine. If I receive 10 leads this month, I would be looking to see how I can get 11 next month. Even if I received 100 leads this month, I want to make improvements so that next month I have over 100.

In this step, I explore the nuances of grading your website and continually keeping it up-to-date in a fast-changing online world. Your website can be your hardest-working employee if you continually train it to do what needs to be done. In Chapter 10 I give you an overview of how to monitor your website for success. Doing this ensures that you can always keep an eye on the goal of your website, thereby improving and enhancing it accordingly. Once you get your website set up properly, it's easy to identify and make changes each month in order to maximize your growth and success.

Principle #6: *Your Customer Determines the Success of Your Website*

• • •

So, there you have it: the three main processes, as well as the six guiding Questions and Principles that I use in the *PT Website Secrets™ System*. This is the tip of the iceberg. Hold on to your hats as we hit the ground running and dive into more detail, more tips, and more life changing advice.

In the coming chapters I give you in-depth information about each of these Principles; we take a closer look at what you need to do to transform your website in order to finally get new patients.

So, what are you waiting for? Turn the page!

5

THE IRONIC SECRET TO SELLING PHYSICAL THERAPY

PRINCIPLE #1: DON'T SELL PHYSICAL THERAPY. SELL SOLUTIONS TO PROBLEMS.

The first principle governing the *PTWS System* is perhaps the most controversial, yet it is also one of the most important. Remember our first question, "what are you selling?" This is the Principle that underscores the answer to that question. It is also the principle I urge you to etch into the fabric of your website: you do NOT sell physical therapy. You sell solutions to problems! It may ruffle a few feathers, and some people may not understand it at first, but I promise you it's one of the single most important lessons you will learn on your road to success.

Let me make my point clear with a little anecdote from my past:

You could hear my creaky rolling walker wheels squeaking down the hall as I approached the patient's room on my left. I reached the doorway, knocked, and was welcomed in by the voices inside. Instantly, my heart sank. It seems like all my patients that day were busy with procedures or too ill for PT, and now I had just walked into a room where a physician was deep in discussion with the patient.

The physician welcomed me in and glanced at my badge - "Christine Walker, Physical Therapist."

"Oh! We are so glad you're here! This patient really needs you!", said the physician.

I was relieved to know that I would be able to work with someone this afternoon. But the conversation degraded quickly.

Glancing at my badge again, the physician exclaimed, "Well that's really funny!"

"What, sir? What's so funny?", I asked suspiciously.

"Well, your last name is Walker and all you do is walk people!", he victoriously proclaimed.

I wish I could say this is a fictitious story, but it's not. It really happened as I described. Apparently I'm a physical therapist and all I do is walk people. And this is humorous because my last name is Walker.

This scenario didn't occur because of my surname, it didn't occur because I was somehow amusing at the time, and it didn't occur because the physician had a bad sense of humor. It occurred because I am a physical therapist.

That having been said, let's take a step back. I know you're a great physical therapist. And I know I am. So, why was my vocation reduced to a poorly timed joke regarding my surname? Because people do not know what physical therapy is; not even physicians do!

The above episode isn't an isolated incident. It happens to almost every physical therapist. Day after day physical therapists are reduced to stereotypes, and they often don't have a platform from which to amend this type of thinking. Why?

DOES ANYONE KNOW WHAT A PT REALLY IS?

It's no secret that the physical therapy profession has long been misunderstood. Most people can't put a finger on what physical therapy actually is, and the strangest part is that most physical therapists can't correct them!

We've all been in the situation where we're asked what we do, and after responding that we're physical therapists, the usual response is a nod, possibly a smile, followed by a vacant expression. Upsetting, isn't it?

We want to believe that people know what physical therapy is. We really want to think that our patients, the public, and the world at large have a great understanding of physical therapy. The problem? They don't.

Let's step away from our years of training and our daily interaction with practical knowledge to think about this from the perspective of the patient. Here's what he or she is thinking:

- Do PTs just stretch people?
- Do PTs just give a few exercises?
- How are PTs different from personal trainers?
- Are PTs just like massage therapists?
- Are PTs just like chiropractors?

These questions are ones which, I think you'll agree, should be easily cleared up. And yet, I'll tell you something very ironic: sometimes the people who have never even been to physical therapy know more than those who've had sessions. Why? Because patients are so seldom informed about what we do. Most physical therapists don't seem to answer their questions.

In my career, I've heard a lot of different opinions about physical therapists from patients themselves. I always ask my new patients what they know about physical therapy, or I ask them to tell me about their previous experiences with physical therapy. And, guess what? The answers are usually not what I expect, and the level of misunderstanding is often surprising.

I've heard everything from the classic, "you do stretching and massage, right?!" to, "I call all PTs 'physical terrorists.'" I've also been told that PT is merely doing ultrasounds and using ice or heat. The bottom line is this: the vast majority of people have no idea what physical therapy is, even if they're a healthcare professional like the physician who thought it was funny that my last name is Walker.

As a consequence, physical therapy is an enigma to most. If you asked ten strangers what it was, you would get ten very different answers. People are generally ill-informed about what physical therapy is, let alone what it can do for their health!

Think about why patients are saying this. Is it because you're a bad physical therapist? No. Is it because no one has ever told them otherwise? Maybe. Or, is it because you never answered their questions on your website? Bingo.

PHYSICAL THERAPY WEBSITES MISS THE MARK

Right now you may be thinking, "but, Christine, my website is so informative!" Well, this is where it gets a little tough. Remember how I told you that each of these principles give you the opportunity to be self-reflective? Think carefully about your website – be open minded and willing to accept that things need to change.

If you do a quick *Google* search you'll see that there are three common types of physical therapy websites all over the internet. You may have one of these websites, or a combination of them, even as I'm writing this. I definitely did when I first started my cash practice, and it was difficult for me to deviate. But, the change was absolutely worth it. Which one are you?

#1: "The Resume"

According to the name alone, you might be able to envision a website that I would call "The Resume". No, it's not a Bourne movie title. It's a type of website on which the business owner tries to emphasize experience, certifications, professional organizations, and any other notable accomplishments. In addition to very detailed biographies of all of the physical therapists and owner, you will also see phrases scattered throughout the "The Resume" website. Example of these include:

"100 Years Combined Experience"

"Excellence in Orthopedics"

"Because Experience Matters"

If you recall, this is a mistake I made when creating my first website. Since I was so young (and definitely didn't have 100 years of combined experience), I felt as if I needed to justify myself and prove to everyone that I was capable of having my own practice only three years out of school. So, I made sure that my certifications and credentials were highlighted.

The problem with this type of website is that the overwhelming majority of patients will not pick your services over another clinic in town based solely on your qualifications. Yes, I realize this is really hard to swallow. If you're like me, you've spent YEARS of your time and WAY more money than you care to admit on your degrees, certifications, and extra training. Of course, we want to be able to flaunt those accomplishments; we want to believe they will get us more patients. But they don't. What patients really want to know is that you're qualified and not a quack with a pretend degree. Beyond that, though, they won't pick you over Joe down the street because you have extra letters behind your name.

Why not? Because they really don't understand what all those qualifications even mean. Let's think about this for a second. When was the last time you understood what the millions of accolades following someone's name meant? And when was the last time you interrogated another professional about his or her academic titles? You never have. Because that never *really* mattered to you. While they may appear impressive, the credentials and training certifications are not going to make you stand out among the physical therapist in your town.

It's a difficult pill to swallow. But, I want you to remember something: your achievements mean SO much more when you have the opportunity to use them instead of talk about them.

Recently, one of my patients confessed how she had picked me over another provider in Charlotte. She said her friends recommended she go see the other physical therapist, but that when she went to his website he only talked his qualifications in dry needling (which she had tried before and didn't like) and ART. At the mention of this last accolade, she smiled and explained that, to this day, she still has no idea what ART is!

She then mentioned how she stumbled across my website. And gratefully, according to her, I didn't talk about any of the confusing qualifications or treatment techniques that really didn't make any sense to her. I wasn't rambling on about my qualifications or special interest in obscure medical techniques. Instead, I talked about runners and how I had worked with them to get them back to running. And, guess what? *That* was all she wanted. So, instead of calling the provider who all her friends had recommended, she called me – and was so happy that she did.

I wouldn't have gotten this patient if I had focused on my qualifications. And the ironic thing is, I actually do dry needling as well, but you won't find many mentions of it on my website. Patients want solutions to their problems – not a journal article about dry needling.

The truth is, you should be relieved to know that your qualifications, or even the treatment techniques you provide, do NOT determine whether a prospective patient will pick you over your competition. Think about that for a second: if that were the case, your competition down the street could take a few follow-up educational courses, grab a few extra certifications, and then be more qualified than you are! Imagine the relentless rat race that would ensue, everyone trying to be the most "qualified." Be thankful that this is NOT how patients make a purchasing decision when it comes to physical therapy! And be mindful of it, too: always turn back to your question – what am I selling?

I'm NOT saying you should avoid putting your accomplishments on your website. You should, but there is a way to do it – one that attracts patients rather than repelling them. If you're interested in how to do *that* then you're going to love one of the later chapters. For now, be aware that a website which is focused solely on your resume is NOT going to generate the massive amounts of online inquiries that you're looking for in order to grow and scale your business.

#2: "The Medical Mishap"

The second type of physical therapy website that you will commonly see is "The Medical Mishap". This is the website devoted to the technical, medical jargon physical therapists deal with in academia. In fact, these types of websites are written by physical therapists FOR physical therapists. It's very common to find that the patient has been altogether left out of their content, and it's even more common for the patient to be entirely clueless as to what's being spoken about.

The thing is, as physical therapists we mingle in tight circles, and that's especially true when it comes to being online. We are used to writing in our 'PT jargon' and speaking like we would to other physical therapists. All too often I see *Facebook, Instagram,* and *Twitter* posts that appear to be directed at prospective patients, but instead could only be understood by other PTs. It is no wonder, then, that the only people liking, commenting, and sharing these posts are physical therapists.

Most of the time, as physical therapists, we talk in a way that other healthcare providers cannot even understand. Yes, that's right. I know this firsthand from my five years in the acute care setting. Most physicians, nurses, and even other rehab specialists don't understand the language we speak in. I had to speak to my professional co-workers like they were patients in order for me to effectively communicate with them.

It really is no different for your prospective patients who are visiting your website.

So when websites say things like:

> *"We provide multiple types of treatment including therapeutic exercise, isokinetic exercise and testing, work hardening, work tolerance testing, manual therapy, dry needling, and pain relief modalities."*

What the patient actually reads is, "we do something very technical which you'll never understand."

When a website follows these technical statements up by saying:

> *"Our goal is to relieve your pain, restore your muscle strength, increase your flexibility, and improve mobility and coordination."*

What the patient really wants to know is, "why and how?"

Given all this, how can we expect any prospective patient to understand what we are saying if we're speaking in technical, academic jargon? Even most healthcare providers, with the exception of physical therapists, would be confused! Why, then, do we expect prospective patients to understand it?

These types of websites are scaring patients away. Can you imagine what they're thinking when they read things like work hardening *(why would I want that?!)* or improve mobility and coordination *(I can already move so, if that's all you do, then you can't help me)*.

I could go on with countless examples; this is so prominent across the internet. Let's be clear about this once and for all. PT jargon, technical lexicon, and academic references should be reserved for a night on the town with your PT friends or for that journal article you've been meaning to publish. In the patient's world, all these garbled, confusing medical terms only confuse the consumer. Joe down the road once again got the patient instead of you.

#3: The "Do-It-All"

The final type of website that I see all too often is the famous "Do-It-All" website. This is the *jack of all trades*, yet *master of none* example I cited earlier in the book. You can do everything, yet you're not showing that you can do anything REALLY well.

In physical therapy school we were taught how to do a little bit of everything. We didn't get taught how to do anything *really well*. That sounds harsh, but as my professor said, physical therapy school only teaches about 5% of what we need to know to be a good – not even great – physical therapist. And this is the standard pretty much across the board. Scary!

The general mentality amongst physical therapists is that, since they teach us a little bit of everything in school, it's easy to assume that we should treat everything. To make matters worse, if you're starting your business, you're likely thinking that you will take any and every patient simply because you're worried about getting as many new patients as possible. I know what this feels likes. Trust me, I've been there.

Yet, this train of thought is what causes people to put words on their websites such as:

> "Our therapists are skilled in treating orthopedic & neurological diagnoses, sports injuries, chronic pain, balance and mobility changes, as well as a variety of other conditions."

Now, take a moment to review that rather broad, longwinded statement. It seems so conflicting, doesn't it? Imagine if Albert Einstein was good at math, science, philosophy, cooking, and the art of fiction, but he was never GREAT at physics... how would we explain relativity? Or, imagine if Nicola Tesla felt as though he was good music, art, calligraphy, and face painting, but he was never GREAT at electrical engineering... do you think we'd be where we are today in technological advancements? The same is true for you – while you may not be Einstein or Tesla, you are REALLY GREAT at what you do. Why not make that clear to your patients?

IF NO ONE KNOWS WHAT PT IS, WHY ARE WE MARKETING PT?

Now that you can spot the three PT website types I do NOT want you to have, it's time to turn to what your website really needs to be. I'll give you a clue... the answer is hidden inside the Do-It-All website mistake. In order to make your website profitable, successful, patient-generating, and sustainable, you need to understand precisely what you're marketing and what you're good at.

To get to that point, let's start with the ultimate question: if no one knows what physical therapy actually is, then why do we market physical therapy all over our websites? In fact, I'll even go a step further: if a lot of people have negative emotions surrounding physical therapy, why are we scaring them away by talking about it on our website?

When you visit most physical therapy websites the first thing you'll see is something about physical therapy. Let's evaluate this scenario. You're a visitor, you have a back problem, and you're desperately looking for information. Yet, once you reach the site, all you see is technical jargon about physical therapy! There's absolutely nothing that will help you.

Here's a little secret: your website only has 7 seconds to win over a prospective patient. I'll discuss this in greater detail in the upcoming chapters, but for now, know that you only have 7 seconds. Is your website able to pique the interest of your visitor in 7 seconds? Probably not. Your visitor is immediately faced with something he or she either doesn't understand or has prior negative connotations about – based on his or her past experiences – so, it's highly unlikely this visitor is going to stay on your website and click around.

Why are we so obsessed with convincing everyone that physical therapy is right for them? What if, instead of trying to teach people about physical therapy, we actually talk to them about how we could help with their problems? The difference is astounding.

To understand why most physical therapy websites flop, you first have to step back and take off your "PT credentials" for a minute. *Most physical therapy websites fail because they think they're selling physical therapy!*

MARKETING <u>OURSELVES</u> VS. MARKETING TO PATIENTS

The idea that we should stop selling physical therapy and start selling answers to problems is a difficult one to get our heads around. I know. My first physical therapy website was all about marketing physical therapy and myself, like so many other PT websites out there. It was a tough decision to change. That's why you still see so many websites focused on benefits such as "excellent service," "1-on-1 care," and "in business 20 years," as if these are the things our patients really want.

Another common trend is for physical therapists to talk about themselves in a way that make no sense to the public. This is the jargon problem cited earlier. Phrases such as, "we're primary caregivers for musculoskeletal problems" and "we provide excellence in rehabilitative care" can be seen on the vast majority of clinics' websites.

And yet, faced with all this, we STILL get frustrated that the public has no idea what physical therapy is. How are people supposed to know what we do from those types of descriptions? Something has got to give.

Remember that people don't really care about us; they care about themselves and their own problems. So, if you can bear with me, eat a piece of humble pie, and read this book, you're going to find out the secrets that 95% of physical therapists don't want to hear (and won't implement). These secrets will give you the opportunity to dominate your town.

Physical therapy has done itself a great disservice by not marketing directly to the people who we, as PT's, help – those people who also happen to be the ones who keep us in business. We're content to market to the doctors, the fitness studios, etc., instead of going directly to the people who actually have problems we can help.

Isn't the reason we fought for direct access so that we can directly reach the people we could help?

We're not reaching those people like we could be. We've created a mess where no one actually knows what physical therapy is! People don't know that physical therapy is one of the best solutions to naturally solve their nagging problems. *We aren't telling them in a way that makes sense.*

We're not in the business of selling physical therapy. Please read that again. You ARE NOT going to succeed if you are selling physical therapy. **Instead, we need to sell the *opportunities*.** For example, the opportunity for a grandparent to play on the floor with her grandchildren again – without worrying about aching knees. Or, if you're in pelvic health, the opportunity for women to be intimate with their spouses again without fear or reservation. Now, that is what people need true help with. And THAT is what you need to sell.

Do you remember the last time you had an agonizing toothache? Did you want to hear about new and exciting techniques in gum research, or did you want the dentist to take away the pain so that you could eat food again? It's exactly the same with your patients. Issues such as a grandparent being able to lift a baby out of the crib so mom and dad can have an hour away from home, intimacy with partners, and even a great golf swing – they are important to your patients. They're so vital that patients would gladly pay for your expertise to solve these problems.

If you want to be successful then *your patients need to see these problems being important to you, too*! If patients feel that the physical therapists are *dedicated to their problems*, then they are comfortable and willing to commit to a plan of care.

How do you instill this trust?

Your website.

If you don't design a website that speaks about the problems your patients are dealing with, then the cycle of misinformation and misunderstanding continues – not to mention you're not getting any business and you're losing money. Without a functional, profitable, informative, and useful website, you'll go back to asking past patients for referrals, emailing Pilates studios, talking to massage therapists down the street, and hoping that the next wave of referrals comes in soon so you can cover the bills at the end of the month. In other words, you won't own your business.

This doesn't have to be the way your business functions anymore. I'm here to show you that, with *PT Website Secrets*™, it's possible to use the internet to directly access your ideal patients, grow your private practice, and get yourself unstuck from this cycle of endlessly waiting for the next referral. **Then you'll finally own your business.**

OTHER INDUSTRIES HAVE THIS PROBLEM, TOO

People are instinctively weary of things that they do not understand. Websites that speak about physical therapy in garbled jargon, about techniques not even other medical practitioners understand, or about qualifications alone, spark fear in the potential patient. No one wants to waste time and money on something they do not understand.

Physical therapists are not alone in struggling to attract new customers online. Another common sector that struggles with bringing in new members via the internet is the religious sector. This might surprise you, but according to the experts who build church websites, the number one thing people want to know before making a decision about which church to try is whether the website shows them what they are supposed to wear.

This may not be that farfetched. When people decide on whether they're going to attend a particular church, their biggest concerns aren't the denomination, the name of the pastor, or even the location. Nope – the biggest concern is *fitting in*.

Fitting in. This is such a fundamental principle to understand. People desire very, very deeply to be part of a community, to be accepted, and to be comfortable. And that is precisely why potential church-goers are dreadfully afraid of showing up to a service and not fitting in. It's their worst nightmare. If a church's website doesn't immediately address this issue, the chance of that church getting new visitors from their online website is small.

In the same way, then, our PT websites need to answer our patients' key questions:

- What will physical therapy do for me?
- How will physical therapy make my life better?
- How do I know this is the right choice for me?

In other words, how do *I* fit in with this physical therapy practice, and how does *it* fit in with me.

WHAT DO WE SELL INSTEAD OF PHYSICAL THERAPY?

We've begun to establish that, instead of selling physical therapy or listing the common conditions you treat on your website, you need to be selling the *solutions to the problems* of your potential patients. The next step is to think about the *type* of problems that you solve.

Here's an example from a business that my family and I love – *Chick-fil-A*. If you visit *Chick-fil-A*'s website, you won't find any mention that "they help people who are hungry for lunch." Yet, of course, they do. They solve this common ailment for my husband, kids, and me fairly regularly. I'm hungry, my kids are hungry, and we need a place to eat – where do we go? *Chick-fil-A!* Yet many places can feed my family, so why do we pick *Chick-fil-A* if we're going out to grab a quick lunch?

Chick-fil-A doesn't sell a solution to my hunger problem. This fact is assumed as a given. Of course, they're a restaurant. If I can pay them to get food, they can make my hunger go away.

Instead of selling me lunch, they sell the fact that it is the perfect place to bring my family. Their allure lies in the fact that they'll greet me at the door and *even* hold it open, will smile while my kids run around and make chaos, and answer everything with "my pleasure" as though feeding me is the best thing ever. Oh, and did I mention that the food is pretty good too?

Instead of selling me lunch, *Chick-fil-A* helps busy moms like me – whose kids are driving them crazy – get the little ones fed, happy, and worn out on the playground so that mom can relax for a bit.

How does this translate to physical therapy?

Most PT websites will say things like, "we can make your pain go away" – yet, that's their only selling point. The problem is, you and I both know that a lot of things can make the pain go away, albeit only temporarily: painkillers, surgery, and maybe even a massage.

Of course physical therapy *can* fix the pain that comes from your knee osteoarthritis, but why choose us over the competitor down the street?

If all you're selling is pain relief, you're going to lose.

If all *Chick-fil-A* sold were lunch, they would lose, too.

You have to know what you are **really** selling, and it has to be something that **customers understand**.

If you confuse, you're going to lose.

TAKE ACTION: *PT WEBSITE SECRETS™ SYSTEM* AND QUESTION #1, "WHAT ARE YOU SELLING?"

[Be sure you've downloaded your free *PT Website Secrets™ System* guide at www.ptwebsitesecretsbook.com/resource so you can plan your website transformation as you read through this book!]

As you're thinking through the *PT Website Secrets™ System* and Question #1 and its accompanying principle, in particular, I want you to think about the following areas in which you can apply the crucial mind-shift needed to market physical therapy:

<u>Orthopedics:</u>

Instead of treating injuries, aches, and pains, you help grandparents become active again so that they're able to get on the floor and play with their grandchildren – without pain and stiffness.

<u>Women's Health:</u>

Instead of treating women with urinary incontinence, you help people who are constantly looking for the next restroom, or those who are afraid to jump on the trampoline with their kids – you help them get control of their bladder and get their lives back.

<u>Pediatrics:</u>

Instead of treating development delay, you help families get their babies moving so that the little ones are back on track with their peers.

• • •

You're not in the business of selling physical therapy. You're selling the transformation of your patient from one situation to another.

You're selling *solutions*! And *that* is what the *PTWS System* is all about – how to reach your patients though the use of a functional, effective website. Once you've made the mind-shift, are ready to make the change, and you're being truly self-reflective about WHAT you're selling, it's time for us to turn to knowing WHO you're selling to.

What are you waiting for? Turn the page!

6

10X THE NUMBER OF PATIENTS YOU ATTRACT

PRINCIPLE #2: IF YOU TRY TO PLEASE EVERYONE, YOU ATTRACT NO ONE.

Driving through the curvy mountains of North Carolina is not the best time to be doubled over in laughter. You really need to have your eyes on the road or else the next bend could be your last.

But here I was, kids in tow, doubled over laughing over the name of a business we just drove by.

Bush Whackers.

This part of my state is known for the beard-growing mountain men, even if a lot of them are college students shielding themselves from the cold weather.

And here, right off the highway, I found a haircutter that had aptly named themselves "Bush Whackers."

Of course, this type of barber would never appeal to me, a woman in her thirties with long, thick hair, but I could instantly see the appeal for the mountain men in town. Of course they would want to go to *Bush Whackers*, and *Bush Whackers* wasn't afraid to call out their people.

With *Bush Whackers'* brazen, courageous name is where our chapter starts. See, *Bush Whackers* isn't afraid to call on the mountain men while sidelining women like myself. They're not afraid to exclude young children, adolescent boys, or teenage girls. Those people are NOT who they're selling to. They're *Bush Whackers* – barbers to the mountain men!

Hilarity aside, this is a super smart business strategy. Yet, it is one that many companies are not willing to implement. What do I mean by that? As a society, we're bombarded with thousands of marketing messages a day – in fact, there are so many that our brains have to tune out 99% of them or else we would be overwhelmed.

The only messages our brains respond to are the ones that really speak to us *individually*, that is, those which stand out from the crowd. Most companies are not willing to take the risk and identify who they best serve and market directly to them. Let's take a few successful companies as examples of this Principle: *Tiffany's* jewelers markets to the upper crust of society, notably women; *Whole Foods* markets to the emerging health-conscious population, notably millennials; *Le Creuset* markets to aspiring chefs, notably those who are foodies. If *Tiffany's* marketed to adolescent boys, the company would fail. If *Whole Foods* started advocating greasy, deep fried cream cheese, the company would fail. If *Le Creuset* began selling their cookware to McDonald's, the company would fail. There *is* success in being a specialty product or service. Remember what I said earlier? Niches matter.

And that's precisely why *Bush Whackers* is such a success! They aren't afraid, and I guarantee that they are reaping the benefits from it.

WHAT DOES THIS MEANS FOR YOUR PT WEBSITE?

This means that you need to start approaching your website from a different angle. The vast majority of physical therapy businesses are not willing to be *Bush Whackers*, and I really want you to be a *Bush Whacker*. Those businesses aren't willing to take the risk and actually market *primarily* to one group of people, and this is particularly true on their websites. How do I know this? Their websites make the huge mistake of trying to prove a variety of skills and abilities, instead of foregrounding a specialty.

Your website must scare some visitors away. If your website is not designed to scare anyone away, then you're not going to have a patient-generating website. It's that simple.

Other industries understand this – *Bush Whackers, Tiffany's, Le Creuset*, the list goes on – yet physical therapists are too attached to the idea of "treating everything" that all too often the people that need help slip through the cracks. Selectivity is NOT being implemented in these business, and it's a big, big problem.

Before you write me off and think I'm crazy, I want to share some stories with you that will show you the importance of being a specialist.

PEOPLE WANT SPECIALISTS

Consider the music industry. Taylor Swift is a specialist at pop/country music. Kanye West is a rapper. Can you imagine the disaster that would ensue if Taylor Swift suddenly decided she was going to take up opera singing? Or, what if Kanye West decided to switch to country music?

What would their loyal fans think? Do you think they would still be interested in seeing Taylor Swift in concert if she was going to sing opera? What would happen to her career and business?

The ramifications of stepping out of their specialities would be huge.

Music stars would never imagine trying to be good at every type of musical craft. Could they make music in different genres? Sure. Would they lose a lot of followers if they started having concerts with five different types of music? Yes.

This principle is true of your physical therapy practice. If you say that you treat everyone, then no one is going to want to come and see you. Why not? Because you must exclude a certain part of the population that needs *physical therapy* in order to attract another portion of the people who need your *help*.

Let's think about that last statement: exclude a certain part of the population that needs *physical therapy* in order to attract another portion of the people who need your *help*. It's a difficult notion to digest. Physical therapy is too broad a concept to market effectively. You absolutely need to narrow down your focus in order to effectively reach those who genuinely need your help.

You might be thinking, "but you've been telling me my qualifications and certifications don't matter! People don't understand physical therapy!" Yes, and I still stand by that. When I refer to specialists, I'm not referring to those people who have specialty qualifications such as, for example, a residency or specialty certification. I'm referring to PTs who market to specific patients for specific problems.

What patients really want is to work with someone *who has solved their problem before*. They don't care if you're a physical therapist, a massage therapist, or a chiropractor. They want someone who has experience with *their exact problem*. That's what gives patients the confidence that they're not wasting their time and money with you.

"BUT I JUST NEED PATIENTS"

The most common, knee-jerk reaction I hear when I share this lesson is: "I just need patients! I don't want to limit who can come see me. I need business!" And truly, I sympathize. I really do. I've been there. In fact, that's exactly how I felt, and how many of my students have felt, when first starting our businesses. But, after working with hundreds of PT businesses across the world, I've come to realize that the businesses that succeed are the ones willing to market to *one single group of people*.

Most cash physical therapy practices fail because they DON'T create their business, especially their WEBSITE, for their ideal patient group.

Remember the Do-It-All websites I previously described? These sites try to be jacks of all trades; that is, the owners market themselves as PTs who can "do everything," thinking that they'll attract everyone to their businesses by doing so. But if you market to everyone, you specialize in NO ONE.

When physical therapists position themselves as the Do-It-All, people assume that you're pretty good at everything, but not **great** at anything. It's the way our brains think. For example, would I be skeptical if my husband's barber told me he also cut women's hair, yet the only people in his barber shop are men? Or, would I doubt it was going to be a good concert if Taylor Swift was set to perform opera, rap, country, and a symphony all in the same concert? Absolutely!

When you use your website to advertise the do-it-all mentality of your business, you are basically telling the world that you specialize in nothing. This is precisely why your business will struggle. Sure, you might get a few extra patients at the beginning, but you will lose 5-10X the amount of patients you could have brought into your business by being a specialist.

FINDING "YOUR PEOPLE"

Since you now see the importance of finding a specific group of people to market to, let's talk about how to actually identify them. This process isn't the same as picking a specialty from a hat – there are a lot of key factors that go into determining who is best to target with your online marketing. I'm here to guide you through the process.

I've already mentioned that your specialty is not going to be orthopedics, neurology, or even pediatrics. These are far too complicated for your patients to understand, let alone to pique their interest. You need something accessible, informative, and directly related to your patients. Thus, your specialty is going to revolve around a certain type of person, instead.

This is a radical shift in your way of thinking: you're moving from PT-centered to patient-centered, and I promise the benefits will be plentiful. The key is to remember that when it comes to marketing ourselves, *we treat people and their problems*. We help them on their journeys to win back their health. We don't focus on diagnoses, which people misunderstand, or are afraid of. Our goal is to make the patient feel comfortable, to build trust with him or her, and to gain his or her unshakable commitment to our plan of care. Therefore, we need to identify WHO it is we are helping so that we can address his or her problems.

How do I recommend identifying your ideal patient group? Take a look.

THERE ARE 4 KEY QUESTIONS TO ASK YOURSELF IN THIS PROCESS

[I've created a worksheet to help you write down your thoughts on these questions. Why? So that you find your ideal patient group! Be sure you've downloaded your free *PT Website Secrets™ System* guide at www.ptwebsitesecretsbook.com/resource so you can record your answers!]

#1: Who do I serve best? Who would I like to see on my schedule all day, every day?

Yes, I do believe that if you're starting your own business, you should take into consideration which patients you enjoy serving. Why shouldn't you? If you love helping these particular people, I guarantee they'll want to come back. Even if this isn't the exact ideal patient group for your website, it's definitely the best place to start.

Ask yourself who you really like working with. Whom do you help the best? I want you to think of actual patients you have worked with in the past, identifying them as people with characteristics, feelings, motivations, and fears.

For example, my ideal patient is a 12 year-old gymnast who competes in competitive gymnastics and who also practices for 20 hours a week. She likes watching *YouTube* and hanging out with her gymnastics friends when not in school or at the gym. Her family is well-to-do with an over $100,000 combined income, and they're seriously invested in their daughter and her potential for collegiate gymnastics. They are willing to do anything to keep their daughter in the gym doing what she loves. But, there's a problem: right now she's experiencing back pain. Her parents aren't sure if it's "just another ache" that frequently seems to surface as part of her sport, or if it could be something more troubling due to its recurrence and intensity.

This description perfectly describes the type of client who I, 1) serve best, and 2) enjoy working with the most. Are you able to describe who you serve best in this amount of detail? I urge you to try. The ability to identify who you serve best – and love working with – is the key to understanding your clientele and being able to market directly to them.

#2: Are there enough of these ideal patients to sustain a business or the caseload that you desire for your business?

This is a vital question. When I first started transforming my website, I debated seriously about whether to "niche down" to gymnastics or stay broadened to active adults and athletes.

At the time, my priority was to grow my cash-based PT business in order to sustain an income that would allow me to quit any other per diem jobs. I realized that there would not be enough gymnasts to fill the number of appointments I needed to see each week. Because of that, I decided to expand my ideal patient to include athletes and active adults.

You'll notice that you could label this as *orthopedic physical therapy*. However, there are a lot of people with orthopedic issues who are not athletes or active adults. If I were to use the technical name, I would be excluding all those patients who do not fit that particular description – and remember, your marketing message on your *website* would be excluding them right out of the gate.

Now that I have two profitable businesses, however, I am shifting my focus back to gymnastics. I only have a certain number of available appointments per week, and I would like to fill them with my ideal gymnastics patients.

This is one of the most crucial business decisions you'll need to make on your journey.

My business coach, Paul Gough, faced a similar dilemma years ago when he opened the *Paul Gough Physio Rooms*. Everyone thought that, since he was a former professional soccer physiotherapist, he would therefore open a sports clinic. But, he took a look at his town and knew he wouldn't be able to grow and scale the business he desired with the population and demographic around him. So, instead of an emphasis on sports therapy, he now focuses on women in their 50's and 60's with nagging aches and pain who are afraid of losing their mobility. He now runs one of the most successful physical therapy businesses in the United Kingdom charging cash while his competition is free.

The question you have to ask yourself is whether you are able to create the business and lifestyle you desire through the notion of your ideal patient. You need to ask yourself whether or not you need to expand your ideal patient population, niche down your ideal patient population, or consider a different ideal patient group. The distinction is crucial, and so is the ability to scrutinize the social and cultural environment of your business.

#3: How can you market to this ideal patient group online?

The next step in finding your ideal patient group for your website is to consider what their online behavior is like. How are you going to market to this population? What media do they consume? Is your ideal patient, or a family member, going to be searching online for solutions to the problems they are struggling with? Where are they going to be searching? Even if you have an amazing website, are you likely going to need to use other means of advertising to drive your ideal patient or their family *to* your website?

You need to start anticipating the online behavior of your ideal patient. Live a day in his or her shoes and try to grasp how, where, what, and when she or he is online. If you have the answers, make sure they are reflected on your website.

If you cannot find the answer and feel as though your ideal patients or their family members aren't reachable online, then you've picked the wrong population for online marketing purposes. That's the time to regroup and be self-reflective. You **must** be able to engage with your prospective patients or their family members *directly* if you want to grow your business by way of your website.

#4: What journey do I take my patients on?

The last important step in making sure you've identified the best ideal patient group is to consider the *journey* your website visitors must take to become raving fans of your clinic. Your website is the starting point – the aim is to hook patients online and THEN get them into your clinic, in person. In order to have an effective, patient-generating website, you must have thought out the process of taking a patient from online inquiry to raving fan.

Here's what this process looks like in *Christine Walker Physical Therapy*:

1. An inquiry, made by an ideal patient, is processed via the website.

2. An effort is made to get them on the phone. It doesn't matter what type of inquiry they've made, my goal is to talk to them and start a conversation about their personal situation. Despite whether or not I actually get the patient on the phone, my follow-up emails are working towards building a relationship.

3. Once on the phone, my entire goal is to get the patient into what I call a *discovery visit*. This is a free 20-minute consult where he or she gets to see my office, meets me, and allows me to investigate his or her problem before any money is exchanged.

4. Based on the discovery visit, I then offer an evaluation. At the end of the evaluation, we agree on a treatment plan and move forward in fixing his or her problem.

This process could take *a week* or it could take *years*. Bringing in cold leads, those people who are less familiar with your business and physical therapy, takes time. Remember, though, it's completely normal.When you're dealing with someone who found you on the internet, he or she is going to need time to grow and trust you before becoming a repeat patient and raving fan.

I have shared this process with you so that you understand the vital role your website plays in jump starting the journey from cold lead to patient. If your website is made correctly, it will attract the clients who are interested, and even excited, in going on this journey with *you*, not Joe down the road.

After all this, where exactly does your website need to lead your ideal patients so that they start the journey of becoming your raving fans? What do they need to see, read, or understand to be willing to take the next step of submitting inquiries, or downloading information, in exchange for contact information paramount in setting up that call?

Keep these questions firmly rooted in your mind as we continue through this book – we'll be taking a much closer look at the areas in which your website needs to transform!

YOU'LL STILL SEE PEOPLE OUTSIDE OF YOUR IDEAL PATIENT GROUP

Just because you identify an ideal patient group DOES NOT mean that you will never ever see anyone outside of that group. You're certainly not barring the doors and using a security guard to chase away ladies in pain if your ideal patient is a middle aged man. Of course not!

When we pick an ideal patient group it's because we're going to focus all of our *marketing efforts* on those people – your website, your advertisements, your blog posts, all of these things will be written **for** them. That doesn't mean you don't want to help others.

For example, let's say you work a lot with youth athletes. It won't be long before their parents start asking you for advice and whether you can help them too. Would you deny their parents the help they need? Of course not! You just haven't orientated your marketing towards them.

Remember, your network of patients will naturally grow via other methods such as word of mouth. I want you to understand that your online marketing, especially on your website, NEEDS an ideal patient group to succeed, but that definitely doesn't mean you will reject others who seek your help.

Don't feel like you're going to be stuck seeing the same person every single hour – it's not true!

WHAT ARE THE IMPLICATIONS OF HAVING AN IDEAL PATIENT GROUP?

Everything you write, design, or create for your website will be done with this specific person in mind. That's a very good thing.

But where do you start implementing the changes? The *About* page. This is the place from which you can immediately make the most impact. In fact, the *About* page is one of the most frequently visited parts of a physical therapy website, second only to the *Homepage*.

I know what you're thinking, though: "didn't you say that my website shouldn't be about ME, Christine?." Yes, I did. But the secret to a successful *About* page is... yes, you guessed it – it isn't actually about you!

Your about page should NOT be used like so many other clinics. Don't put a laundry list of diagnoses and/or treatment techniques online. All too often, prospective patients land on an *About* page only to find their fears confirmed: you're not really a specialist, you see all kinds of people with scary diagnoses that are indecipherable on your website, and you do all sorts of weird treatments that don't make much sense to them. Yikes. You're not going to convert those patients!

If you want someone to scan and barely look at your *About* page, then by all means, list every diagnosis and treatment technique you've seen or used in the past five years. But, if you truly want to appear as the expert in solving problems people want answers for, take down the diagnoses and treatment techniques right now.

Instead of listing common conditions and treatment techniques on your website, you need to be talking about **who you really help**, **who they really are**, and **what problems they're really struggling with** in their lives. The *About* page needs to be used to establish a connection with your ideal patient group so that they feel extremely well understood.

Are you doubting this will work? Let me give you an example from my own website:

On my clinic's website you won't find any mention of ankle or foot pain (except maybe if you dig deep in the blog). It's not there. There's no list of conditions I treat.

Instead, all over my *Home* and *About* pages (before I converted my website to be only for gymnasts) I talk about athletes and about how I treat various sportspeople, including runners. I talk about how I can help get them back to the sports and workouts they love. And guess what? I get tons of runners with foot pain. One month in 2018, every single one of my new evaluations was a runner with foot pain.

When I ask these patients why they inquired after my help, their answers are always the same: "you talked about runners and getting them back to running. Everyone else talked about stuff I don't understand."

And these responses prove that it's that simple. It's not that all the other physical therapy businesses can't treat foot pain, and it's not that my patients don't know that, it's that the other physical therapists' websites don't connect with their visitors... so they lost patients to *someone who had a website that did – someone who was willing to risk talking to a specific population.*

THE BRUTAL TRUTH

When I published my first website it was hard not to have a sense of pride. I now had my own company and I was able to proudly display all my accomplishments and credentials, all of which I had worked very hard for AND spent a lot of money on. I naively thought that because I was on the internet, I had "made it" – and that made me feel validated.

While it made me feel really good, it did not make potential patients feel any better about what they were going through. That's because *they* are as self-focused as I am! When someone is in pain, or struggling, what do they like to do? Talk about themselves and what they're going through.

And if your website isn't giving them the information they need, they're going to look somewhere else.

In this chapter I have shown you how important it is to know WHO you are marketing to on your website. I've shown you that to be brave and to speak directly to your perfect patient group – even if that means sidelining others – is a huge leap towards business and financial success.

I've also indicated that the do-it-all mentality is a sure-fire way to stunt your business growth. Remember, if you are good at everything, how can you possibly be GREAT at anything? Marketing a specialty – a particular problem that you can solve for your ideal patient – is one of the single most important things you can do for a successful website and a successful business.

So far we've established WHAT you need to sell and WHO you're selling to. Are you ready for the next Principle? Let's get ready to find out how to make sure your visitors PAY ATTENTION.

I'm excited, are you? Turn the page!

7

YOU WILL
LOSE IF YOU CONFUSE

PRINCIPLE #3: PEOPLE DON'T PAY ATTENTION TO (OR BUY) THINGS THEY DON'T UNDERSTAND

We've established that you need to know exactly WHAT you are selling and WHO you are selling to – but, how exactly should you grab the attention of those visiting your website? For that, we need Principle #3 – people don't pay attention to (or buy) things they don't understand. As we move through this chapter lodge this idea firmly in your consciousness: if you want to be successful, you need to grab attention via a website that has understandable, relevant content. This is vital! Here's a story that shows exactly what I mean:

John Davidson thought he had hit the jackpot. His first website, which he launched for his fitness gym, was working. It was bringing in consistent new gym members and helping grow his business. So, he decided to have the same web developer build his cash physical therapy website. If his gym website worked so well, wouldn't the same format and content work for his physical therapy business?

He dished out a lot of money to have the web designer build a site for his PT practice. The design was the same. All he changed was the words and pictures to reflect physical therapy instead of the gym. It seemed like a foolproof idea.

Fast-forward one year, and lots of money and frustration later: John realized that his physical therapy website was a complete flop. It wasn't doing anything to bring in more new patients for his fledgling physical therapy practice. In fact, one new patient told him that she almost didn't call because she looked at the website and thought she needed to be fit in order to come to his PT clinic.

As a result, John knew something was very, very wrong. In the wake of the success his gym website produced, John had wrongly assumed the same type of website would best serve the interests of his PT practice. Exactly the opposite had happened; he was losing money and, worst of all, he was scaring potential patients away! Something had to change, and that's when John reached out to 'PT Website Secrets™' for help.

With the help of *PT Website Secrets™*, John came to understand that marketing physical therapy is not the same as marketing for gym memberships. The clientele in each sector have different expectations; they are looking for different information when shopping online for perfect solutions to their problems.

In John's case he didn't consider one simple difference. When people are looking for a gym to join, they have a general idea what they're getting, which is a place in which to work out and get fit. But, when people are looking at physical therapy they are completely confused about what they are buying into. And it is John's job to clarify that!

His first PT website did the exact opposite. On the one hand, John's gym website was covered with amazing photos of young men and women lifting weights. It appealed directly to the exact clients he wanted to attract. Why? Because that's what his potential clients wanted to see when they were looking for a high-intensity bootcamp-style gym. Truthfully – and this is absolutely key – it didn't really matter too much whether he put pictures or words on his website. Why? Because people had an idea of what they were buying.

His physical therapy website, on the other hand, also had pictures of his ideal client exercising – yet, these pictures didn't attract his ideal PT patients. Why not? Because those people still had no idea what physical therapy was by looking at pictures of fit, young people in a gym.

Now, I understand John's thought process: he figured that the people visiting his PT website would see the pictures and realize that he will help them get back to doing what they love. Unfortunately, that didn't work. There was simply no information or content that was answering the questions those people needed solving.

Because John was relying on his pictures to tell a story and to give his potential patients information, he was losing patients daily. These pictures were not telling visitors more about his services or what he could do to solve their problems. In consequence, John was getting zero enquiries from his website, and this is indeed a very bad place to be.

There is a happy ending! A few months later, after having his website transformed by *PT Website Secrets*™, he's now getting consistent calls from potential patients. And better still, he constantly hears things like, "I found your website and knew you could help me." Isn't this a wonderful thing to hear as a PT? His business is booming, and guess what... it all started with the transformation of his *Homepage*.

THE MOST IMPORTANT PAGE

Many people know that the first page of your website, known as your *Homepage*, is the most important page on the entire website. But, many people do not understand WHY. What's the end result? In other words, what makes the *Homepage* so important, and how should it be used in order to maximize its impact? There are a lot of amazing looking, professionally-styled *Homepages* out there, yet they do nothing to grow businesses, get more new patients, or get the owners home in time to tuck their kids into bed.

Why is your *Homepage* so vitally important?

Because you only have seconds to capture someone's attention and keep him or her on your website.

It doesn't matter how much time or money you've put into making or designing your website. The success of your website, and thereby your physical therapy business, hinges on your ability to capture the attention of your ideal patient group in merely a few seconds.

GOLDFISH HAVE BETTER ATTENTION SPANS

In 2015 *The Times* published an article titled, "You Now Have a Shorter Attention Span than a Goldfish".

The article explained that goldfish are notorious for having a very short attention span – nine seconds, in fact. Yes, that's very short, but the article then continued to reveal an even more surprising fact. A recent study in Canada by *Microsoft* revealed that since the year 2000, when mobile and hand-held electronics exploded, the attention span of a human dropped from 12 seconds to a mere eight seconds!

The title is humorous and humbling all at the same time. If we're honest with ourselves we know our attention spans are diminishing. While scary, if you want your business to succeed, you need to be very clear on this.

We're bombarded by thousands of marketing messages a day, all of which are trying to get our attention. Our brains can't handle it all. Our minds get overwhelmed by trying to filter out what's important and what can be forgotten.

This is something we all experience 0 daily, only sometimes it's more obvious. Think of the last time you went shopping for a big ticket item like a television. Were you overwhelmed by the amount of choices and features available? Did you have trouble figuring out which things you needed and which things you didn't? Of course. It's the name of the game.

The theory is that as people use various types of media *at the same time*, like watching television while browsing on your phone, people are having an increasingly difficult time filtering out irrelevant information. While we're getting better at multitasking, we're also getting worse at paying attention to what we're doing.

And this is a problem for you. Why? Because you're a business owner trying to grow your company through online methods. While prospective patients are using the internet to find solutions to their problems, they're also paying less attention while doing so.

What are the implications of this for your website?

Well, you have to have your *Homepage*, particularly the part "above the fold", perfectly structured in order to have a chance at attracting new patients via your website. What exactly do I mean by that? Keep reading to find out!

HOW TO BEST USE YOUR 7 SECONDS

"Above the fold" is a term taken from the newspaper industry. It used to be commonplace to purchase newspapers from newspaper stands – something our internet-loving population probably doesn't relate to anymore. On these stands the newspaper was folded so that you could only see half of the front page.

Newspaper sellers quickly realized that they must put their most eye-catching and interesting headlines on *this* part of the paper, above the fold, in order to get the most sales. The term is now being applied to websites – our online version of the newspaper. What you see when you land on a website, without scrolling, is considered "above the fold." Of course, keep in mind that, since a website is a dynamic media, this could look different on various sized desktops, mobile phones, and tablets.

Many physical therapy websites, even as I write this book, are losing hundreds – maybe even thousands – of new patients. Why?

Because they do not have their websites designed properly above the fold.

Looking back to the research from *Microsoft* regarding attention spans, and observing our own highly distracted behavior, we can confidently say that you literally have a few seconds to capture the attention of your ideal patient with your website. If you don't grab attention in the first couple of seconds you risk potential patients hitting the dreaded back button and going to your competitor's website.

HOW TO GET WEBSITE VISITORS TO PAY ATTENTION

Like a successful newspaper, the best way to get a visitor's attention on your website is by using the space above the fold to speak directly to your ideal patients, their problems, and how you help people exactly like them. Similar to the newspaper, a headline, rather than a picture, is the best way to accomplish this feat.

As the previous chapters have shown, pictures do very little to convert potential patients, let alone to truly grab their attention. The visitors don't understand the pictures, and they're not informative enough to truly hook interest. Pictures do attract attention, but for the wrong reasons, and, as a general rule, pictures don't attract paying clients.

PEOPLE BUY BASED ON WHAT THEY READ, NOT WHAT THEY SEE

Once again, we need to turn to the nature of our own behavior to understand why prospects make decisions about physical therapy businesses; decisions which are most often based on what they *read* instead of what they *see* on your website. Here's an example:

A few years ago our dryer broke and it was time to shop for a new one. I went online to look at new dryers. Did I buy the first good-looking dryer that I saw? Nope. Did I actually care what the dryer looked like at all? No, I did not. Did I read about all the specifications and compare prices before purchasing? Yes. I made a decision on where I would purchase my next dryer based on what I read on the websites, not based on how flashy the company's website looked. No amount of pictures displaying shiny new dryers would make me buy one; only information would.

Amazon is a great example of this. If you look at *Amazon's* website, it's not particularly pretty. It's hideous compared to a lot of other businesses in the industry. Do you know what *Amazon's* website really is? It's simple and practical. It has all the information I need to make a decision about whether I want to do business with *Amazon*. They make it so easy to purchase that it's a no-brainer.

If *Amazon* is doing this, you should, too. *Amazon* customers are practically identical to your own potential patients: they want answers to their problems. If *Amazon* isn't flashing strobe lights and displaying elaborate pictures, why are you?

When patients are looking for a solution to back pain, they're not looking for the place with the coolest pictures. They're looking for proven solutions that specifically cater to people like them; solutions that will get them back to doing whatever activities they prioritize in life.

In other words, they will make a decision about your physical therapy business based on what they read on your website.

THE PICTURE PROBLEM

If you recall my personal story in Chapter 1, I bought into the lie that the best physical therapy websites have the best pictures – this couldn't be further from the truth. With my first website, I spent hours wasting my precious time on design elements that weren't going to make a difference in the number of patients I received as a result of my online presence. Little did I know at the time, but pretty pictures and logos are not what makes your physical therapy website successful, and they certainly don't help you grow your business.

The scary thing is that pictures may actually be deterring website visitors from calling your practice. Pictures are very powerful, but they are also very subjective and can be interpreted in many ways. One of my clients had a video of a guy canoeing on his clinic's *Homepage*. Sounds pretty idyllic, except that his clinic was landlocked in the middle of a state nowhere near a body of water on which to canoe. How many people do you think landed on his site and hit the back button because they thought they were in the wrong place? A lot. Within 24 hours of revamping his old site, he had a new patient from the internet for the first time. And there were no pictures of canoes or any other sporting activity to be found anywhere on his website.

THE CLEAREST MESSAGE WINS

The website which uses the space 'above the fold' to speak clearly to their ideal patient group is going to win – not the website with the coolest pictures above the fold. You need to spend a significant amount of time on perfecting your website's message above the fold.

So what should sit above the fold on your website? The headline.

The headline is the first set of words that someone sees when they land on your website. It should be a simple phrase or sentence that clearly defines *who your physical therapy clinic best serves* and *what you can help them accomplish in their lives.*

These words should be tailored precisely for the ideal patient group you identified in the last chapter. In order to be effective, the best headlines rule people in, rule others out, and make the targeted ones feel like your business is perfect for them. Remember, if your headline doesn't turn some people away, then it won't attract anyone either.

At the time of writing this chapter, here is what you can find at the top of my website:

"We help active adults & athletes in Charlotte, NC get back to the workouts and sports they love without injections, painkillers, or multiple trips to the doctor's office."

Within several seconds you know exactly **who** I help *(active adults and athletes in Charlotte)*, **what** I help them accomplish *(get back to the workouts and sports they love)*, and **how** I help them avoid the things they don't want *(injections, painkillers, or multiple trips to the doctor's office)*.

Every part of my headline was designed with my ideal patient in mind. I created it and modified the words based on what my ideal patients tell me when I work with him and her. I also tested the words on my patient population multiple times, trying different words until it worked for my website and started attracting my ideal patients.

People will try to copy my headline – or even my entire website! – and not get the same results. The reason is that their ideal patients will never be exactly like mine. They haven't worked with my exact ideal patient and they won't understand why I used the particular words in this sentence.

Only *you* know your ideal patient group. The goal is for you to understand them better than they understand themselves. If you can do that, then you can craft a headline that will entice them to stay on your website for more than a few seconds without being distracted by the latest *Facebook* or email notification.

With the above headline, I hook the exact patients who are best for my business. They will explore my website below what they immediately see when the website loads.

If the headline doesn't speak to you, then you'll know you're not in the right place and I will happily encourage you to hit the back button. This has two positive impacts. First, it makes my ideal patient feel more special and as though they're in the right place, and second, it is the first step in filtering out patients that are not a good fit for my business and would be a headache to deal with anyway.

CLARITY IS KEY BELOW THE FOLD

Now that we have captured the attention of our ideal patient group, we need to look at the strategy for the rest of your *Homepage*. **Clarity** is the secret key to furthering the relationship with a website visitor as they explore below the fold.

Once the headline has done its job and attracted your visitors' attention, it's time to approach the the rest of the *Homepage*. At this point in the relationship, the website visitors know that we work with people like them to solve their problems, but they're still extremely skeptical. After all, this may be the first time they've interacted with our brand and their collective knowledge of our services is limited.

When you first go to a website that you've never looked at before and the headline captures your attention, what do you do next? You quickly scroll through the rest of the *Homepage* to see if something else will capture your attention or affirm that you're spending your time wisely. Remember, attention span quickly fades in a matter of seconds, and we therefore risk the likelihood of a distraction which would take our visitor's attention away.

Let me tell you a secret: everyone **scans** *Homepages*. This means that your *Homepage* must be scannable. Here are two common mistakes that I see physical therapists make:

Mistake #1: The *Homepage* Is Cluttered

There is so much text on the front page that you would think someone is writing a novel. What's wrong with giving so much information? At this point your website visitor is looking to gather *quick bits of information about your business*. He or she is not interested in reading about every single detail that you have to offer. A cluttered *Homepage* is information overload for their brains, and instead of paying attention they start to tune you out. Remember, they're bombarded with messages all day long, and if something isn't clear and easy to understand, then they will overlook you. The patient is looking for further confirmation that he or she is in the right place, and moreover, that he or she might find some useful information on your website.

Mistake #2: The *Homepage* Is Almost Empty

I'm sure you can think of many websites with *Homepages* that contain only a picture and perhaps one line of text. There's no ability to scroll and there is a very limited direction as to what to do next on the website. Don't be fooled into thinking that this will get visitors to start randomly clicking around. When people land on these types of websites, they get confused. They start thinking, "what do I do next?", "where is all the information?", and "how do I find what I need?" People prefer to be guided into what to do next. When they land on a *Homepage* with virtually no information, they feel like they're awkwardly walking into a party where they don't know anyone and have no idea what to do or who to talk to.

YOUR HOMEPAGE IS YOUR MOVIE TRAILER

The only time I go to the movie theater is once a year for the new *Star Wars* film – I grew up on *Star Wars* and absolutely love everything about the franchise. Between two kids, two businesses, a husband, and a dog, I barely have enough time to watch a *Netflix* show on my own sofa.

The idea of planning, finding a babysitter, and blocking 3 hours out of my day to go to the movies is overwhelming. In other words, I need to be insanely hooked by a movie trailer to actually take time out of my busy schedule to go see it in a theater.

Yet, that's exactly what happened to me in 2017 when I was at the movie theater with my husband to watch *The Last Jedi*. Before the movie began, I saw a trailer for *The Greatest Showman*. I was instantly hooked. The music, the story, all of it captured my attention, and I knew it was the type of movie that would be best experienced on the big screen. I wanted to see it...desperately.

Have you ever seen a movie trailer that captured your attention so much that you knew you were going to have to see it? Maybe for you it isn't movies – perhaps it's the latest smartphone, your favorite musician's album, or even the latest book in a trilogy. Was the teaser for the product was so enticing that you instantly wanted to know more, read more, and get more information?

Your *Homepage* is your movie trailer. It gives you the opportunity to do a powerful thing: preview the offers and ways you can help people in a simple and quick manner, thereby peaking curiosity and making visitors want to know more.

The impact of a powerful *Homepage* is tremendous. If you can ignite interest in your website right off the bat – so that visitors stick around and browse longer – then not only are you furthering the relationship and increasing the chance they will become patients, but you're also going to be rewarded by search engines like *Google*. Yes, that's right! When you get someone to stay on your page, click around, and browse, it tells *Google* that your information is **useful** and *Google*, in turn, will reward you in the search results.

THE PRACTICAL IMPLICATIONS

The entire goal of your *Homepage* is to guide people and to help them decide what to do next, to either *take action* with your business or *learn more* about your business. We want to make it **so** easy for them to figure out how to do business with you that they practically don't even have to think about it.

Your *Homepage* is not supposed to reflect anything and everything you do as a business, and more importantly, it's not supposed to be about you. For a *Homepage* to be successful, it needs to:

- **Call out those who you best serve** and *turn away* those who are not right for your business. (*PTWS* Principle #2)

- Instantly **introduce solutions to problems** that your ideal patient is struggling with. (*PTWS* Principle #1)
- **Introduce offers with clarity** so that people know what action to take next. (*PTWS* Principle #3)

The great news is that with a clear, targeted headline above the fold, and functional, clear information that is scannable below it, you can accomplish all 3 of the above criteria.

Now that we've covered the importance of the *Homepage* in terms of grabbing attention, it's time to turn to how to craft offers. In order to run a successful website and business you need to have offers which *meet* your visitors in their decision-making processes, thereby helping them to take the vital steps towards your business and away from your competitor.

If you're ready to learn how to make the perfect offers, join me in the next chapter.

8

HOW TO GET WEBSITE VISITORS TO TAKE ACTION

PRINCIPLE #4: PEOPLE WON'T TAKE ACTION UNLESS YOU ASK

Let me start this chapter by saying that I happen to love pizza. It's by far my favorite food and I really do think I could eat it every day if it weren't so unhealthy. that wasn't an extremely unhealthy choice for my body. While I usually make my own pizza at home, occasionally we do order delivery. Some nights, especially when you're a mom, you need a pizza delivered, STAT!

When it comes to pizza, I'm pretty simple. Pepperoni makes me very happy and satisfies my deepest pizza desires. Lately, I've been venturing into some other combinations, mainly adding feta, parmesan, and tomatoes, but no matter what I add, I always come back to my tried and true favorite – pepperoni.

It's clear that I love pizza, and given my love for the tasty fast food, you wouldn't think I'd hesitate to pick up the phone and call for a pizza. It's simple, right? Dial the number, give your order, and get your pizza thirty minutes later. But to me, however, the experience is far from simple.

When I get on the phone with the pizza place, I typically get put on hold – and I don't know anyone who likes being on hold. Then, when it's finally time for me to order, I have to scream over the commotion going on in the background of the pizza store. Usually I'm asking the employee to repeat my order, simply because I'm sure there is no way he or she heard me. There's a decent chance my pizza will be delivered with the wrong toppings or even in the wrong size.

As a result, I spend the next thirty minutes in anxious anticipation of my favorite meal, hoping that it's going to be right. If it isn't, we're going to have very unhappy kids and a very unhappy mama.

Here's where you fit in. The beautiful thing about the pizza ordering business is that, since pizza stores got smart and started using their website or smartphone apps for ordering, I no longer have to have the stressful, frustrating ordering ordeal.

Instead, I can quickly hop on my phone or computer, punch in my order without being placed on hold and without background noise, and be assured that my order was placed correctly and will be delivered by a certain time. It's magical, and it makes ordering pizza a joy instead of a chore.

Do you want your potential patients shouting over background noise, praying that they get the right treatment, hoping that you were able to understand them, and that you actually care about them at all? Of course not. You want them to *love* doing business with you. And that's exactly what your website can help you achieve!

YOUR POTENTIAL PATIENTS HAVE THE SAME FEARS AND DOUBTS

Keep in mind that your prospective patients are having the same fears and doubts about the experience of going to physical therapy as I do about ordering pizza on the phone. It might sound strange, but it's true.

Unfortunately, no matter how great your customer service is, your patients have been scarred by hundreds of previous frustrating customer service experiences. So much so that their expectations are incredibly low and they doubt whether they really want to call you, even if they know they need physical therapy and really want it!

This situation desperately needs to change.

TWO CATEGORIES. TWO DIFFERENT STRATEGIES.

I'm going to give you two different strategies for tackling the problem of hesitant potential patients. Your website really can help you convert them. Here's how: generally speaking, when prospective patients visit your website you can split them up into two categories: cold leads and warm leads.

Cold leads are those people who are beginning to learn about your business, are highly skeptical, don't trust you, and are seeking more information. They are really not sure what to do about their problems, or they may even doubt that there are any real solutions to their problems. They aren't ready to take any action or admit they have problems, but they *are* trying to understand their current situation, desperate to gather information on what to do next in order to placate their concerns.

They are searching online for information, using search engines like *Google*, free online help from videos on *YouTube*, reading blogs and other informative articles, and are downloading free resources. They are not yet ready to commit any money towards fixing their problem. At this time, they're looking for advice and will be scared away by pushy sales pitches.

Approximately 85% of website visitors will fall into this category. But don't fear – we're going to talk about how to nurture this group into warm leads in the next chapter.

Warm leads, on the other hand, are those patients who know they have problems and also know that physical therapy is a possible solution for their issues. They are actively seeking the best physical therapist to solve their problems and get them back to the things they want to do. They are looking at different physical therapy websites online, comparing the messages on each website, and trying to make a decision on who they are going to contact.

Approximately 15% of your physical therapy website visitors will fall into this category, and in this chapter we're going to talk about how to design your website in order to have the best chance of getting this group of people to contact your business.

The key point is that your website will need to cater to both groups, and to do that successfully you will need elements that focus on **both** cold leads and warm leads. In other words, you need to make both groups feel comfortable, informed, and supported.

Let's start talking about what you need to do to get the warm leads – those who are actively seeking physical therapy – to actually contact your business after they find your website.

WHAT WARM LEADS WANT

In the story at the beginning of this chapter, I talked about how I love pizza, could eat pizza all the time, and yet still dread picking up the phone to call and order a pizza. Why? Because of the experience I anticipate. The key word is **anticipate** - whether or not the experience is as I imagine, I have on occasion not ordered pizza because I didn't want to deal with the *hassle* of ordering it.

Your potential patients have the same fears and doubts. They may want physical therapy, and even want to work with you, but they may not be able to pick up the phone call you. They have busy lives just like you! The idea of being tied up with someone on the phone, or the worry of being placed on hold for minutes on end, will keep them from actually calling. And yet, all too frequently, the only option I see on a physical therapy website is for inquiries to "call now"!

If we want to capture the 15% of warm leads that are truly interested in doing business with us, then we need to give them options. Every warm lead isn't going to be attracted to the idea of "book or call now." They may be highly interested in physical therapy, but have a few questions that they need answered first.

Asking them to "call now" makes them feel forced into a decision, because they have no other choice. If you offer multiple options of how they can start a relationship with your business, such as ask about availability or talk to a PT on the phone, they are more likely to take action because you are speaking to their personal desires and meeting them where they are in the decision-making process.

MAKE DOING BUSINESS SO SIMPLE THEY CAN'T RESIST

In my coaching program, one of my students told me how excited she was to get a particular new patient. He was a busy executive and fit her ideal patient profile completely. He told her on the first visit that he never would have picked up the phone to call, but since her website gave him other ways to inquire about appointments, he was able to start the process in the middle of a business meeting.

The lesson to take from this story, as well as my pizza ordering analogy, is that *the business who makes it the simplest will win.* When designing or transforming your website you have to make it so simple to do business with you that it's a no-brainer for the potential patient. Otherwise, you'll have visitors landing on your website, only seeing the option to call, and hitting the back button because they either don't have time or are scared to pick-up the phone and call even when they know they need help.

THE SOLUTION ISN'T WHAT YOU THINK

The solution to this problem is NOT online scheduling. In fact, I'm a fierce opponent of online scheduling for first-time clients. Before you stop reading, I completely understand your hesitation.

I know the idea of online scheduling for new patients is very attractive, especially if you're a solo practitioner without a secretary. Cutting out a phone call and avoiding the game of phone tag – where you're trying to get someone on the phone at the right time – sounds super appealing, but the truth is it's too good to be true.

Having new patients schedule online is all about convenience for the physical therapist, as opposed to that of the new patient. This method of scheduling puts up a barrier between yourself and the new patient.

How many new patients do you know have booked an appointment without asking either the secretary or the physical therapist a single question? I can't think of any in my multiple years of being in physical therapy. People always have questions, doubts, fears, concerns, or at least want to hear the voices of the people they're going to be working with. It's human nature. We want to start building relationships and gaining familiarity – remember what I said about *fitting in*? No one likes to show up when they are completely unfamiliar with their surroundings.

Online scheduling for new patients is about the *convenience*, not the *experience*. And that is definitely not what you want.

What do I propose instead of online scheduling? Multi-step forms.

FUNCTIONAL FORMS

Multi-step forms are an absolute asset to your website and future patient conversions! It's true. I love simple web-based forms for many reasons, but without a doubt they've had the biggest impact to drive my business forward and get new patients via my website. Here's why:

First, forms are easy to fill out and can be completed in less than a minute. That means a busy executive, or even a mom of three kids, can complete such a form without the hassle of interrupting their schedules. Think about how many people you are losing from your website because they don't have – or think they don't have – time to pick up the phone and call you.

In lieu of this, many clinics will tell me that their alternative to "call now" is to say "email us." If we're thinking about the same types of people who don't have time to call, do you think the idea of sitting in front of blank email is more appealing? It might be more terrifying – they will worry about things such as the quality of their writing or the information they give. This scenario does not make the potential patient feel comfortable in the slightest.

Forms solve this problem by providing a template that walks them through their current situation, their problem, and what information your business needs in order to determine if you can help them. In this case, the website visitor doesn't have to think much. They answer a few simple questions about their situation and they're done.

Forms not only *simplify* things for the consumer, but they do the same for the physical therapy business. They are easy for the secretary or physical therapist to review quickly, and they contain all the information needed to make a first phone call to the prospective patient. These forms are a win for both the website visitor and for the business.

THE MULTI-STEP MAGIC

When I first added forms to my website, it was a complete disaster. No one filled them out. Why? Well, I tried to "simplify and save" by using the forms that I could build through an email provider, which was Active Campaign at the time. My simplification was actually one long page consisting of 8-10 visually intimidating, uninviting questions. Not very functional or comfortable. To be honest, my first form looked like I was asking my visitors to write a memoir, not give me necessary, clear, easy information.

Like so many other elements of my website when I first created the forms, they got absolutely zero entries – people didn't fill them out or ask about my services. As you know by now, I don't give up when something is a complete failure. Instead, I analyze the puzzle and try to figure out how to make it work. If other business owners could get multiple forms filled out by their ideal patients each week, then I knew I could too!

My first step was to switch from my novel-style forms to be multi-step. Instead of being visible on a single page, the 8-10 questions were divided between multiple pages. Why do that? To make the forms look *less intimidating* to complete. Now they appeared simple, easy, and inviting.

In fact, this change gave my website visitors the opportunity to tell me their stories quickly, highlighting their main concerns and how they were impacting their lives. After this, I could then ask for their personal contact information at the end.

After changing to multi-step forms, the number of forms being filled out skyrocketed. I had tailored the form in a way that my ideal patient would appreciate, and as a consequence they were happy to fill them out! Now, instead of worrying about when the phone will ring, I receive to new inquiries from forms being filled out on my website at all hours of the day.

The other amazing thing about adding forms to your website is that it extends your office hours. Website visitors feel like they can interact with your business and start the process of doing business with you anytime, even if they're lying in bed at 2 A.M and unable to sleep because of their pain.

Adding multi-step forms to your website will also cut down on the amount of people you lose to forgetfulness, those who *plan* to call you in the morning, but then *life gets busy* and they forget. It will give your business the opportunity to engage with prospects on all days and at all times.

Here's the truth: the 15% of website visitors who are ready to do business with you, but for whatever reason cannot pick up the phone at the exact time they think of your business, absolutely love multi-step forms. And that's precisely why you need them!

GIVE THEM OPTIONS

The other secret to successful multi-step forms is to not have one, but to have at least 2-3 different ones, thereby offering alternate starting points for your warm leads. For example, on my website at the time of writing, I offer three different forms that can be filled out:

1. Ask About Availability and Cost
2. Talk To a PT on The Phone
3. Free Discovery Visit

The funny thing is that these forms are not significantly different, only their titles are! The strategy behind this is recognizing that my ideal patients are in different legs of their journeys, and that different offers, therefore, will be more appealing than others. When I present multiple offers I increase the chance that something is going to resonate with the patients personally, and increase the chance that they click on one and fill out a form.

If I only offered a "Free Discovery Visit", it would guarantee that I won't capture the entire 15% of warm leads. There are plenty of people who have no interest in a free visit, but instead have questions and would like to talk to a physical therapist on the phone.

Other warm leads will primarily want to know about availability and cost of treatment. For them, the corresponding button is going to speak to their thoughts *exactly* and entice them to submit their information.

Either way, the entire purpose of the forms is to get the business relationship started, and, as a result, get their contact information.

These three options are ones I have tried and tested on my ideal patients. These are the options that they want. Your ideal patient may want something similar, or something entirely different. The key is to think about your ideal patient's journey and what they need to make a decision about physical therapy.

THE GOAL IS TO GET THEM ON THE PHONE

While this may seem ironic, the entire goal of offering different multi-step forms is to get the prospect off of your website and onto the phone. The big difference you experience with the forms is, instead of asking them to jump the entire river at one time, you're laying down stepping stones for them to get across the river and onto the phone.

For example, take one of my best students, Jennifer McGowan. She's a busy mom of 4 children and also a solo clinic owner. She needed a website that would be working for her 24/7, one which would capture leads even when she was busy with taking care of her family.

After taking the *PTWS Workshop,* she transformed her messaging and implemented the 3-step form strategy on her website. Since then, she's been getting 12-15 hot leads per month from her website...without having to take extra time away from her children. This has dramatically grown her business in the 6 months she's been open! What would 12-15 new hot leads who are interested in booking physical therapy do for your business? How about for your lifestyle?

While the website captures the information of these leads who are ready to buy, it doesn't completely eliminate all communication with the potential patient. You and/or your staff will have to speak to warm leads at some point. It's foolish to think that your website can completely replace the power of human-to-human interaction. Instead, your website is there to bridge the gap and to help initiate the first human-to-human conversation.

There will always be questions to answer and things that the prospect wants to know – and apart from your website, you, the therapist, lay the *foundation for the experience* with your business during that first phone call. And *that* is why it is absolutely vital your multi-step forms drive your potential patients to this point.

YOU STILL HAVE TO ASK

The 15% who are warm leads want to do business with you, but the crazy thing is that you still have to *ask* for them to do business with you. Why? Because if you don't ask, they're going to assume you're not confident enough in the service you provide.

This is not the time to be passive-aggressive, *suggesting* that people should, for example, "fill out this form if [they] want to." Instead, this is the moment that you confidently say, "if you're looking for physical therapy and want to know how we can help, call us or fill out a form now – it will only take a few seconds."

This comes back to our busy lives and the thousands of marketing messages we hear/see each day. We will always filter out the marketing messages that are not confident in their offers or that don't actually tell us what to do. We're so overwhelmed with information that we have a hard time making decisions – we need to be guided into exactly what to do next. Once again, you need to make it *so easy* to do business with you that no one who is a warm lead could ever dream of hesitating.

The warm leads are the ones we want to speak to directly, those whom we confidently tell what to do next, and those whom we follow-up with quickly and regularly. The growth potential for your business from this one website strategy is **huge**. If you can successfully determine what offers your ideal patient is attracted to, and create multi-step forms related to those interests, you will capture the warm leads visiting your website.

Understanding your ideal patient, using multi-step forms catering to their needs, being confident in your service, and willing to guide your ideal patients to that vital, relationship-building phone call, will take your business to new, unimaginable success. Remember, make it as easy as ordering your perfect pizza online and ditch the blaring noise, the confusion, and the anxiety.

Now, it's your turn. How many warm leads are you missing out on from your website simply because you're not giving them enough options for how to do business with you? Keep that in mind as we move on to the next chapter, where we'll discuss how to entice, keep, and convert cold leads into warm leads through the use of your website.

Are you ready? Let's go!

THE PROFIT IS IN THE PURSUIT

PRINCIPLE 5: REVENUE RESULTS FROM REAL RELATIONSHIPS

Have a careful look at the essence of Principle #5: *you need to pursue and nurture a relationship in order to convert and keep potential patients.* This is such an important part of your journey to success that I want to reiterate this with an example. Take a look:

Imagine for a moment that you're limping down the street, grimacing in pain as you desperately hold your back in an attempt to find relief. Seeing this, I approach you and say, "HEY! I'm the best physical therapist in the world and I can cure your back pain! Want to be my patient?" How would you feel? How would you respond? And would you jump at my offer?

Of course not. You'd probably be very freaked out, and I imagine you'd try to quickly brush me off and say, "no, thank you, I'm fine," even though you're clearly NOT fine.

Why was my hypothetical approach so wrong? It's intimidating, for one. And secondly it doesn't make the potential patient feel comfortable at all. He or she doesn't know me, what physical therapy is, or how I can help. Everything about this scenario makes alarm bells go off in his or her head.

Unfortunately, this exact interaction is how most people feel when they visit physical therapy websites. Visitors are often bombarded with an onslaught of promises, which to them seem empty and unsupported, and, understandably, they're a little freaked out. Why? Here's the key: because *we fail to establish authority* and *trust* before asking for someone to "call and book now!"

All too often PT websites make the mistake of failing to consider that our ideal patients are at different stages in their journeys at the time they encounter our website. Some are warm leads and some are cold leads. And these two groups of leads are distinctly different in their interactions with your website.

Remember, cold leads – the 85% who are not ready to take immediate action – are definitely not in the same phase of their journeys as the 15% of warm leads. In fact, some of the 85% might still be wondering if they really have a problem. They don't know if they need you, why they need you, or what you can do them for them. And that is why nurturing good relationships with them, building trust, and making them feel secure, is absolutely vital for your business' success.

How do we begin doing this? Let's outline the different types of people who fall in the 85% of cold leads to get you started:

PERSON #1: COMPLETELY CLUELESS

This is the first type of person you'll find in the 85% of cold leads. These people are completely clueless and don't even know they have a real problem. Generally, they assume that the pain they are experiencing is completely normal and that everything is okay.

A great example of this is found in women's health. So many postpartum moms assume that having pelvic pain and bladder leakage is normal after birth; they don't even realize that something is wrong and so they are not looking to do anything about it. It's only when they come across information about their conditions that they are made aware and educated about the irregularities of the symptoms. It's at this point that they begin to realize they have a situation that needs to be addressed.

For you to reach these types of people, you have to give information that addresses their specific problems. Remember the chapter about WHO you're targeting? Your patients need to be given information that will ignite their consciousness, meaning they will start realizing they have problems you can help them with. And the best way to do this is to make sure your website speaks directly to them!

PERSON #2: FORGET-ABOUT-IT

This is the second type of person you will encounter. The forget-about-its are aware that their bodies are not working properly, but mentally they are not in a place to deal with the situation. They're ignoring the warning signs in their bodies and hoping the pain or problems will go away. Many people in this stage are in denial before realizing that the problem is only getting worse.

How many people live with pain on a daily basis, but don't actually do anything about it? I bet you've even done this yourself! You wake up one morning with an ache and hope it will go away. Before you know it, you've been waking up for over a year (or more!) with this same pain.

In my family, it was my dad. He waddled around for years with bad knees but didn't think he had the time to actually do something about it. Instead, he powered through for years, despite being immensely uncomfortable. This is a prime example of someone who is trying to "forget about it" and is not yet ready to address the fact that something is wrong and that it needs attention.

The key is to realize that because someone is in pain, doesn't mean they're ready to solve their problem.

This is such an important part of your PT business, especially when it comes to your website. It is human nature to feel pain and to hope it will disappear. We, as PT's, understand that physical therapy is the best way to deal with the problem, but we also need to understand that the patient might be in a state of denial.

Sometimes the patient might have to go through a mindset shift, and get to the point where he or she decides that enough is enough. This is the point at which he or she will take action and consider your business. You need to support them right from the start, all the way through their journey to this point – and your website is the perfect platform to do this.

Remember, many people will browse online for days, weeks, or even months looking for the right person and service that resonates with them. In order for your business to stand out, your website should be spurring people on to take action. Your website needs to guide these types of visitors into a proper understanding of their problems, why they need to start taking care of themselves right now, and why YOU can help them.

PERSON #3: THE DOUBTER

The doubter is the type of person who knows he or she has a problem, but what holds him or her back is the nagging doubt as to what to actually do about it. These people aren't ignoring the issue like the forget-about-it group. Instead, they are actively seeking a solution, yet are having trouble making a decision about what is the best thing to do.

Many of the fears a doubter has come from being burned in the past. Have you ever made a decision that turned out poorly? Of course you have, and it's safe to assume that you're fairly skeptical about trying a similar thing again. The reality is that many of our ideal patients have been sold miracle treatments that haven't worked. They've wasted time, money, and probably endured even more pain in the process. Whether it's the latest fad product for back pain, or another healthcare provider or alternative practitioner – even another physical therapist – the pain of making a wrong decision PREVIOUSLY will incapacitate your ideal patient's ability to decide what to do next.

The fact that they've tried other solutions in the past, which have all failed, will hold them back from reaching out to your PT business and asking for help. It's a vicious cycle that they get stuck in!

Without certainty that your physical therapy solution will solve their problems, these doubters are likely to drag their feet and wait for long periods of time before reaching out to your business.

In order to get doubters to become patients from your website, you have to instill the belief that you have successfully solved problems like theirs in the past. You must gain their trust in your ability to help them.

PERSON #4: THE EXCUSER

Excusers know that they have problems, and they even know that physical therapy can help, but what keeps them in the 85% of people who won't immediately take action on your website is the immense amount of excuses getting in the way.

For the excuser, his or her health is not the highest priority. They'll drag their feet even when they know physical therapy can solve the problem. These people are more concerned about things such as time and money. They don't prioritize getting the solution to their problems, and this is keeping them from taking action on your website and getting help.

In order for you to help the excuser, you must educate him or her on what he or she needs to prioritize. You need to educate him or her as to their problem and WHY they need to take action now. And the best way to do this? Your website!

PERSON #5: The 15%

Though not strictly part of the cold lead group, the remaining 15% - warm leads – are worth mentioning one more time. As you'll remember, these people know that they have problems and they're ready to give physical therapy a try. They take immediate action on your website by filling out forms, picking up the phone, or getting in contact via online methods such as live chat.

The biggest goal of your website is to move persons #1 through #4 closer to becoming the 15%. And that's exactly what I'll show you how to do in this chapter.

IT'S ALL ABOUT TRUST

By now I think you've come to understand that a big part of converting and keeping potential patients is building a relationship of trust and security. All of the scenarios above ultimately come down to one thing: a lack of trust.

The primary reason someone will not deal with your physical therapy business is a lack of trust. The overwhelming majority of visitors to your website – approximately 85% – will not be ready to do business with you because they don't trust you. Should you give up on these people and only go after the 15% who are ready to solve their aches and pains? NO!

It's going to be really hard to grow a business if you're only focusing on the 15% in the last chapter. You'll have some success for a short amount of time, but after a while you'll hit a plateau and not be able to grow any further. You need to expand your focus to include the 85% of people who are not yet ready, and you need to make them ready.

Your business's survival and growth will depend on your willingness to pursue the 85% who say no to you the first time. That means you have to change your mindset in order to grow the successful physical therapy practice of your dreams.

Instead of thinking that "no" is a negative response, you have to think of it as "not yet." The vast majority of people need multiple touch points with your business before you will gain their trust. It's not about never, it's about when.

HOW TO GAIN TRUST

It used to be said that seven or eight touch points were needed before someone would do business with a company. By touch points I mean moments of interacting with, or learning about, the company. This could be via an advertisement, a download, a workshop, a phone conversation, a visit to your website, a video, or many other activities. Today, with an increase in skepticism and increased reliance on crowdsourcing opinions, this number has grown closer to ten to fifteen.

Touch points help build trust between you and your potential patients, and as such, they help maintain a relationship that will eventually lead to a conversion.

In the previous chapters I talked about how we don't even take our friend or family's word for things anymore, that we naturally go online to do our own research before visiting that restaurant or going to that doctor. Your potential patients have the same exact skepticism about you. They don't trust you (yet). That's precisely why you need touch points.

You must think of your website as the relationship starter. Most consumers have too many options, and this results in decision fatigue. It becomes hard to pick a specific option because you're not sure which is right and you don't want to make a mistake.

The problem with most websites is that they don't start a relationship that builds trust between the business and customer. Most PTs wrongly assume that having a professional-looking website, and showing off credentials, will increase trust. But that's just talking all about yourself! Imagine if you went on a first date and talked only about yourself – there's a good chance you're not getting a second date! Other people are just as self-centered as we are – and this definitely doesn't exclude our potential patients.

Your website and your entire business is for your patients. Touch points make this abundantly clear, thereby instilling trust, comfort, security, and at the end of the day, conversions to paying patients.

HOW TO USE YOUR WEBSITE TO ESTABLISH TRUST

So now that you know how important building trust is, how exactly do you do it? There are 3 key ways to use your website to establish trust:

#1: Free Valuable Offers
#2: Social Proof
#3: Expert Information

We're going to spend the rest of this chapter diving into these 3 strategies, but before we get going, I want you to notice something very important. On my website I have many different options, all with the purpose of developing a relationship with my visitors in order to establish trust. In this way, I increase my chances of having something available for every single individual who's an ideal patient. And this is what I want for you.

TRUST BUILDING ELEMENT #1 – FREE VALUABLE OFFERS

Free valuable offers are known in the marketing world as "lead magnets." A lead magnet is simply a freebie download that you give away in exchange for a prospect's contact information.

You've probably seen these on websites you've visited. You might even have downloaded a few. They're everywhere, and they should definitely be on your PT website. They are popular for one reason: they work! Internet users are happy to give their email – and even phone number – in order to have a download they want.

Examples of lead magnets could be free guides, a quiz, an audio or video mini course, or anything you can send in exchange for someone's contact information.

On my website, at the time of this writing, there are free downloads with more information about the main specific problems that I see in my clinic, and importantly, the problems that my perfect patients are searching for on the internet. However, certain problems are searched for more than others. One of the biggest mistakes I see is people offering downloads for problems that their ideal patient is not readily searching for online. Make sure you understand your ideal patient group and are offering something that they see as valuable.

Another important thing to realize is that you don't have to offer free downloads for every diagnosis that you see. In fact, you will get more downloads if you limit yourself to 3-5 free download offers! Why? Because otherwise people will get overwhelmed, distracted, and have a hard time choosing how to start a relationship with your clinic. You want to make this as simple as possible. Stick to at most 3 to 5 free downloads on your website.

Offering lead magnets on your website is critical, because there are a lot of website visitors who you would never have an opportunity to follow up with if it weren't for the contact information you receive in exchange for the free downloads. It's really hard to start a relationship and establish trust when you can't get in touch with someone!

These freebies are perfect for the 85% who are still information-seeking and are not yet ready to take action on their health problems. They are downloaded because they have more perceived value than "free" information that is readily available online like a blog or article. Please read that again. Downloads have a higher perceived value, and they will be taken more seriously, than information that can be easily obtained without downloading.

To successfully use freebies in order to attract the 85%, you must make sure you know your ideal patient group very well, so that you can offer them exactly what they're looking for.

When a prospect opts-in to one of my offers, I gather his or her contact information. My website has officially produced a result that will grow my business. I now have the phone number and email address of someone who needs my services in my area. My website has accomplished its mission! And I want this for your website, too!

TRUST BUILDING ELEMENT #2 – SOCIAL PROOF

Another powerful way to gain the trust of the 85% is by social proof, also known as testimonials. When used properly, testimonials build trust and confidence while simultaneously positioning you, the physical therapist, as the expert.

Website visitors need to see testimonials in order to believe that you're not an online hoax. Remember, the doubt and distrust in your business is very strong at the beginning of the relationship. Testimonials go a long way in bridging the gap. The nice thing about them is that they can come in different forms, from quotes to stories told by text or via video.

Different types of testimonials need to be used in different places on your website. On your Homepage we must keep testimonials scannable, meaning they need to be simple and no more than a few words or a sentence long.

Your website visitors do not want to read or watch a long testimonial on your Homepage. That will scare them away! They won't read or watch it. Period. So on your Homepage you need to pick a few quotes that are easily scannable and have powerful words of affirmation. That way, when the website visitor scans your homepage for the first 5 to 7 seconds, they see positive words about you and start having positive associations with your business.

On the other parts of your website, including where you're offering free downloads, you can give longer text or video testimonials. Your ideal patients will relate most to the testimonials that are told in a story form: problem, solution, result, future.

The best testimonials initially talk about the problem that the client was struggling with and what prompted his or her decision to finally seek help. Then, a great testimonial transitions into talking about what solution finally solved the problem and what the end result was. At the end, the strongest testimonials look to the future and talk about what life will look like now that the problem is fixed.

With the problem, solution, result, future model in mind, it's easy to look at your current testimonials and find which ones are best at helping you establish social proof and increase trust.

TRUST BUILDING ELEMENT #3 – EXPERT INFORMATION

Another excellent way to establish trust and start building a relationship is by giving away expert information for free and without requiring an opt-in. Some of the 85% will be so skeptical that they will not want to opt-in for anything from you, at least not until they learn more about you and your business.

Why should you give away so much free information in order to get someone's contact information? Although you may know you're an awesome physical therapist and a trustworthy person, the potential patients who land on your website are immensely skeptical of you. It's very, very likely that they've been unsuccessful with other bad advice in the past. They're scared to death of making the same mistake.

WHY YOU MUST GIVE TO GET

The purpose of all this giving is to establish trust. If I'm willing to give so much information away for free, then what I offer as a free download, or even a paid service, must be amazing!

A fantastic way to give free expert information is by establishing a blog on your website. This is great not only for the 85%, but also for your *Google* search results.

On my website you can find a blog with tons of free articles talking about common problems I see in the clinic. I use this space to answer frequently asked questions from my current patients. You can also read more specifically about common injuries that people have, such as back pain, neck and shoulder pain, and knee pain. At the end of most blog posts, I typically repeat a free download offer. Oftentimes someone is willing to read more and give their information afterward.

One of the fastest ways to establish trust is by being willing to give away something before asking for anything in return.

ARE YOU IN?

Most physical therapy business and their websites are built with only the physical therapist in mind. In other words, they aren't built for the 85%, and many aren't even built for the 15%!

The physical therapy businesses that are willing to do the hard work of building and nurturing relationships with the 85% are the ones that grow, scale, and end up finding the financial and time freedom they've been looking for in business all along.

This process starts with the website, which is the online foundation for your entire business. It's your place for your people. **It's your online domain.**

Transforming your website to speak to and capture the 85% is only for those who are willing to work and build a powerful, functional, relevant online domain. Are you in?

If this is you, and you're ready to take your PT business to new heights through the use of your website, join me in the final chapters of this book as we go through the actions of your visitors, the next steps, and how you, too, can start scaling your business via your website, right now!

What are you waiting for?

10

HOW TO DETERMINE
WEBSITE SUCCESS

PRINCIPLE #6: YOUR VISITORS' ACTIONS DETERMINE THE SUCCESS OF YOUR WEBSITE

As we're coming to the last chapters of this book, I want to tell you something very, very important: building your website is not a one time deal. Thinking this way is perhaps the worst mistake a physical therapy business owner can make. Assuming that once the website is built then nothing else has to be done has been the downfall of many a PT business.

If you're not willing to continue to monitor and make changes to your website and online presence on a weekly basis, you might as well put down this book and forget all about predictable lead generation via an online presence, and you can forget about being a successful business owner. If you think this way, stop right now and save yourself the time and money you'll invest in building a patient-generating website.

Building your website is not a one time experience. Please re-read that. Your website is NOT done and dusted once you've done your initial overhaul. Building or transforming your website is just the beginning! At the end of a website transformation, there's only one way to determine if your website is going to help or hamper you; there's only one way you can be 100% sure that you've **gotten into the Owner's Club**, a place where you can predictably generate new patients, on your own, from the internet. Your customer has to tell you.

HOW DO YOU MEASURE A WEBSITE'S SUCCESS?

If you cast your mind back to Chapter 1, I told you that in the beginning stages of my business I mistakenly assumed that my website was amazing simply because other friends, family members, and physical therapists told me so. Even as I was anxious about money and where my next patient was going to come from, I was content to live with that website simply because I assumed it wasn't the problem. I did this for over a year because other people told me it was great! What I didn't know at the time was that my first website was the biggest mistake holding back my small cash practice from massive success. I can honestly say that, looking back now, I am so thankful I changed my website and changed my life.

As a new physical therapy business owner, it's easy to be persuaded by the wrong advice. Don't be hard on yourself. The mistake is made in good faith and for good reasons. We are trained as physical therapists, not as the CEOs of companies. We think like physical therapists, treat like physical therapists, and even talk like physical therapists. Therefore, many of us rely on outside advice for the "business matters" early on in our career. While this tactic is not inherently bad, many of us take advice from the wrong people, especially regarding our websites.

IT DOESN'T MATTER WHAT PEOPLE THINK. WHAT MATTERS IS WHAT THEY DO

Throughout this book I have explained that your PT website is the backbone of your business. It is the engine running your marketing, your conversions, and your reputation. It sets you apart from other PTs in your area, and it gives you a distinct edge over your competition. It is also your first port of call when it comes to sales, and that is why I can confidently say that in order for your business to succeed, you have to start thinking like a CEO.

In your case, your website's success, and as a result the success of your business, depends on the ability of your online presence to KEEP YOUR IDEAL PATIENT in mind at all times. How will you know whether you're succeeding? By monitoring what your ideal patient actually does with your website!

It' not about what everyone thinks. It's about what your ideal patient thinks.

Your ideal patient, or even your friends and family, may think your website is average in appearances, but remember that people don't make business decisions based on appearances. They only take action if the website speaks directly to them about their situation and solving their problems. No one is paying valuable attention to pictures that make no sense to them. And NO ONE is going to act on a picture that doesn't speak to them, help them, or solve their problems.

This is kind of how I feel about my car. I'm not a huge fan of my car's looks. It has been pretty beat up by my kids, my dog, and especially me over the past 12 years of its life. But, I still drive it happily from one place to another because it's trustworthy, reliable, and gets done what I need it to do.

For my clinic, it doesn't matter what my friends, my fellow physical therapists, or even my husband thinks about my website. I don't care. It sounds harsh, but in order for me to be successful, I need to care about whether or not the active adults and athletes take a step closer in a relationship with me and my company after visiting my website. And I do! I wonder... did they fill out a form? Did they take a download? Did they read the blog content? Even if the visitor isn't my ideal client, maybe they know someone who is? Do they forward the website to a friend who needs it? These questions aren't vanities, they're very real ways of how I want and need my ideal patients to interact and take action on my website.

Your website's goal should be the same. You shouldn't care what people say about its looks, and you definitely shouldn't make changes to the website based solely on opinion. You should only gauge your website's success on whether or not it causes the people you are trying to reach to take action with your business. You have to start asking these types of questions while keeping your ideal patient in mind. It is the single best way to know whether you're successful.

Your website should never be a stagnant, finished product. It should be a working, living, functional, targeted arm of your business. YOU own your business, and YOU are making the decisions. After you've transformed your website using the previous five *PT Website Secrets*™ Principles, asking these question and being self-reflective means that you have truly joined the Owner's Club. You're a true owner. With that power comes a responsibility: now that you've reached Principle #6, you have to constantly adapt, test, and monitor your website by observing the interactions of your ideal patients.

THE LIFELONG JOURNEY... MASTERING PRINCIPLE #6

Mastering Principle #6 comes down to your commitment to monitor, either on a weekly or monthly basis, what is going on with your website and where to make adjustments. One of the worst mistakes PT business owners make is to set up a new website based on the fundamental *PTWS* Principles and then not look at it for a year. You **cannot** build a website just to leave it unattended!

You would never go through the process of hiring a new employee and then never train them. The process is continuous for as long as he or she is with you. Why? So that you can constantly improve his or her performance for your company. It's like teaching your newborn all you know before age one and then naively expecting them to grow up into a responsible adult! Why would you leave your newborn website to its own devices?

Your website can be your hardest-working – and cheapest – employee, but only if you continually train it to do what needs to be done, similar to any other employee in your company.

What exactly do you need to monitor, and how do you go about getting started? First of all, there are many different numbers that you need to monitor on a weekly basis in order to gauge the changes that are required on your website. I could – and perhaps I will – write an entire book on this topic in the future. For now we'll lay a foundation for understanding the basics.

MONITORING YOUR DASHBOARD FOR WARNING LIGHTS

The *PT Website Secrets™ System* of building a website is strategically designed to make it simple and easy to monitor your website. The *PTWS System* gives you specific indications of whether changes need to be made. In my signature online course, the Workshop, I teach clients how to build websites so that they can monitor each of these individual metrics and **truly know** whether their websites are working for or against them. Think of metrics as a series of warning lights similar to those on your car dashboard. They tell you that something might be wrong and that it is time to look deeper into what's going on. Here are the three main warning lights you need to be tracking:

Warning Light #1: Number of Visitors

You have to know exactly how many unique visitors are landing on your website each month. If you don't know how many people are visiting your website, you can't figure out what the problem is. If you build a 5-star hotel in the middle of the desert, but no one knows about it, is it a bad hotel? Or is it a good hotel in a bad location? If no one is finding your website then you can't determine whether or not your website is working.

You may have a fantastic website, but due to inactivity you start believing it's a complete failure. Not so! The problem is that you don't have enough website visitors. The number of visitors must be monitored first so that you can make educated decisions on where changes are needed. It's kind of like making major treatment decisions based on one case study in a medical journal. You'd never do that. You need a larger sample size. If you have less than 100 visitors a month, then you may need more visitors before deciding what is and what is not working on your website.

Warning Light #2: Tracking The 15%

If you've exceeded 300 visitors a month, it's time to turn to where changes should be made. You need to find out how many of the 15% are taking action. This means that you have to have an eye on how many forms are filled out on your website, as well as the number of phone calls that come into your business because of your website.

Tracking these numbers requires a coordinated effort between website statistics and talking to your front desk team, or, if you're a solo practitioner, evaluating all the calls you've taken personally. Make sure your team is asking callers where/how they chose to call your clinic!

Warning Light #3: Tracking The 85%

To determine whether your website is building relationships with the remaining 85% of potential patients – those who aren't ready to take action, yet – you must track the number of people viewing and downloading your freebie offers. Tracking both aspects of these numbers is crucial, as it helps you identify where any disconnect could be occurring. If a lot of people are viewing your freebie offer page, but aren't opting into the offer, then there is most likely a disconnect between what the offer page is promising and the message on the opt-in box.

So, by keeping a consistent eye on these three numbers will give you a lot of insight into where your website needs adaptations. Remember, the internet is always changing. Our habits on the internet are evolving. One offer which may speak well to your ideal patients this month may fade the following month.

Think about television ads – even those for the biggest companies. They're constantly changing. Why? Because smart marketers know that the same offer won't work forever. That's why advertisers are always coming up with new ads! We wouldn't take action and do business with companies if we saw the same ad for years. So, don't let your website become stagnant!

Warning lights are there for a reason, and I urge you to monitor, enhance, change, and adapt your website constantly. Your website is for your ideal patient, and everything you do, write, post, explain, and offer is for him or her. Always keep your website on track by using him or her as your guide.

· · ·

In my clinic, my website is my greatest ally – it brings me consistent, dependable patient generation, gives me invaluable data about my business, allows me to spend quality time with my family, ensures that I reach the people I most want to help, gives me financial success, and perhaps most importantly, gives me peace of mind. Gone are the days of hustle-style marketing and working 14 hour days to pay the bills. With my *PT Website Secrets™ System*, I have been able to break free and truly embrace the dream I have always had: being a real owner, a PT who helps those she cares about most, and a business owner who OWNS HER BUSINESS, not the other way around.

If you're ready to learn how you, too, can become the true owner of your business, join me in the final chapter of the book as we discuss how to get into the Owner's Club!

11

HOW TO GET INTO THE OWNER'S CLUB

There you have it, the only system you will ever need to make your website your hardest working, most profitable employee. The *PT Website Secrets™ System*, with its 6 overarching Questions and Principles, is your path to the freedom, financial success, peace of mind, and life you have always dreamed of. And with the tools to monitor, alter, and change your website from the get go, you're set to achieve unbelievable success.

In the last chapter, I pointed out that learning how – and being willing to – switch up your website based on the actions of your website visitors and your ideal patient is the key to climbing the ownership mountain and achieving Owner's Club status.

Remember, **whoever owns your traffic, owns your business.**

If you're reliant on word of mouth referrals, then your customers own your business. If you're reliant on other referral sources such as physicians, fitness studios, gyms, massage therapists, etc., then those professionals own your business. Your business's success or failure is intimately tied to the success or failure of those other people – you don't own your business!

You only own your business when you can predictably self-generate new patients ON YOUR OWN with direct-to-patient marketing – and the only way to do this is via your website!

If you can do this, you've made it. You've achieved your dream of being a TRUE physical therapy business owner, and you've hit the pinnacle of success known as the Owner's Club.

Once in the owner's club, you won't have to hustle for referrals or worry when the next new patient will be coming in. Your website will be consistently converting website visitors into new patient leads for your physical therapy business.

Here's the *Ownership Mountain* again. Where are you?

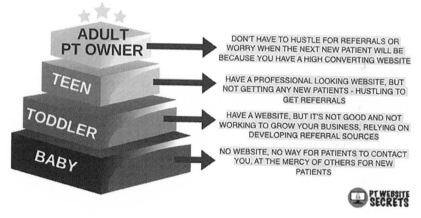

More importantly, where do you want to be on the *Ownership Mountain*? Are you at a stage in your journey where you're 100% committed and finally ready to break free from your dependence on others, thereby TRULY owning your business?

If you've made it this far into this book, then I know you are truly serious about finally owning your business by transforming your physical therapy website. I know you're ready to give up going to bed at night worrying where the next new patient is going to come from. I know you want to gain that online advantage over your competition and make the most of the opportunity to market directly to your ideal patients online, a move that will make them happy to pay your fees and become life-long customers and raving fans. I know because I am one of you.

The *PT Website Secrets™ System* has worked for hundreds of physical therapists like you from around the world. The strategies in this book have been applied to all types of practices, including cash-based, out-of-network, hybrid clinics, and even the traditional insurance-based clinics, all with wild success. This system works. Period.

The *PTWS System* has been so successful that at least one of my PT Website Secrets™ clients has used the strategies to add $40,000 extra revenue to his business in one year!

Do you remember Kris, my first clinical instructor in PT school, whom I talked about in Chapter 2? Seven years after being his student intern, the tables turned and Kris came to me for help with his website. He had moved back to his hometown of Lexington, KY, had started his own private practice, and was about to open a second location.

His business was doing okay, but his website was doing nothing to grow his business. He was completely reliant on doctor's referrals or word of mouth. With his second location opening, he worried whether he would be able to fill the new clinic's schedule.

Kris built his first website with help from his wife. The site was more or less an online brochure that said "we do physical therapy," had a few pretty pictures, and some staff bios. There really wasn't much to it.

I took Kris through the *PT Website Secrets™ System*, and together we identified his ideal patient, identified what he was selling, crafted a unique headline, created offers for the hot leads (the 15%) and the cold leads (the 85%), and transformed his website.

Within 3 months, Kris was getting 1-2 new patients from his website each week. He was so excited he called to tell me that he did the math and over the year this small jump in new patients would conservatively add at least $40,000 to his patient billing. What would $40,000 do for your business this year?

HOW YOU CAN TOO

I want you to experience the success, joy, stress-free lifestyle and financial freedom I have come to achieve using the *PTWS System*.

Since you are a serious physical therapist, a CEO-minded individual who's ready to transform your business, who is committed to becoming a confident and successful business owner, then I believe you are very likely to benefit greatly from diving even deeper into the *PT Website Secrets™ System*.

For this reason, I want to invite you to join me in free live training where we can dive deeper into the *PT Website Secrets™ System*, thereby transforming your website to be a patient-generating machine. This is additional free training and is the logical, best next step after this book. Go here to access the free training: www.ptwebsitesecretsbook.com/training.

I've seen physical therapists grow their businesses TENFOLD simply by implementing the *PT Website Secrets™ System*, and all that in less than a year! These physical therapists are finally physical therapy business OWNERS; they've escaped the hustle-style marketing that wears us all down – and forced me onto bedrest with my second child. My greatest desire is for you to escape the same hustle of running around chasing referral resources – I want you to generate new patients by marketing online directly to your ideal clients, and, in so doing, I want you to **join the Owner's Club ASAP.**

I created the *PT Website Secrets™ System* so that you could get more people to see that the physical therapy you provide is the solution to their problems. We both know how much you can impact their lives for the better, and it's time they knew, too. I learned early on in my career how few people understood what physical therapy actually is, and yet, I also realized that the majority of those people needed physical therapy to live their lives the way they wanted. But they didn't know it. That's heartbreaking! It's time your website started telling them.

I COULDN'T KEEP THIS TO MYSELF

When I set out and risked my time and money to learn all of these strategies, I never thought I would be sharing them with you. I was concerned about the survival of my own business and dreading the idea of going back to work for someone else after maternity leave.

Once my website was transformed and consistently bringing me new patient leads, I realized I couldn't keep this information to myself. There were too many other amazing physical therapists having the same struggle to get patients who desperately need their help off the internet and into physical therapy.

I've shared my story and all the information that I spent hundreds of hours and thousands of dollars to learn. Why? So that you can see it's possible to transform your website and **own** your business.

You can achieve freedom from financial and time constraints so that you, too, can spend more time with your kids, spend more time with your patients, and go to sleep at night knowing your website is working for you 24/7 to grow your business.

Together, using the *PT Website Secrets™ System*, we can help more people who desperately need the services we can provide to change their lives. We can do this by building websites that truly help our ideal patients make better decisions about their health, something that few other physical therapists are willing to do. We can do this by NOT marketing physical therapy.

Many circumstances in my life have reminded me of how limited my physical abilities are, and the reality that I can only treat so many people each week dawned on me over time. Maybe you're facing the same reality, either because of a full schedule, or, like me, an unpredictable health problem. By helping other physical therapists transform their websites and OWN their businesses, we can reach so many more people who need physical therapy desperately but don't know it.

As physical therapists, we're all about helping people, but without the proper website, we handcuff our ability to impact our community for the better – this holds us back, both personally and professionally, from the dreams of owning a business and building the life we desire. We're stuck running around, appealing to other business owners for referrals, and unable to grow our business or get home to tuck our kids in bed. The *PT Website Secrets™ System* is the #1 process to escape the hustle trap and get your business noticed by your ideal patients.

WHAT IF YOU DON'T?

My greatest desire for you is to take everything I've taught in this book and use it to transform your website and your online marketing, so that you can finally start owning your business and generating new patients with direct marketing.

The *PT Website Secrets™ System* is all about building relationships with people who desperately need your help. It's about serving your community and the people around you with your God-given skills as a physical therapist. If you keep on doing what you're doing now, something which isn't bringing you much joy or financial success, then you're missing out on your chance to greatly impact the people around you.

Sadly, I see too many physical therapists who play it safe. They're content to do the safe things: read books, listen to podcasts, and take a few courses. They do all these things passively, never actually committing and taking action on anything they learn. Coincidently, then – or perhaps not – these are the business owners who feel stuck and claim that nothing works.

If you don't take action, nothing is going to change. Please re-read that. The current methods you're using to market your business online are not working. You're still reliant on other people for your business to survive. You're still hustling to find new patients from other referral sources instead of marketing directly to your patients. The reality is that you aren't going to get higher up the Ownership Mountain without making a change.

Unfortunately, the majority of you who read this book won't take action after finishing it. But, for those select few who are truly serious about their businesses, I really look forward to hearing from you and celebrating your results! Be sure to send me your story at christine@ptwebsitesecrets.com.

THE OPPORTUNITY

If you are one of the few who is determined to take action and make a change in your business, I want to invite you to work personally with me, Christine. If you're interested, you have two options on what to do next:

<u>Option #1: Free Online Training with Christine</u>

The *PT Website Secrets*™ online training is a free, in-depth webinar that shows you the key changes you must make to your website to finally get new patients from the internet. (Sign-up at www. ptwebsitesecretsbook.com/training) I show you exactly how my most successful *PT Website Secrets*™ students have gotten into the Owner's Club and are currently predictably generating new patients for the physical therapy businesses without the hustle of marketing to other referral sources.

In the training you'll see how everything we've talked about in this book gets implemented on successful websites. You'll get to learn directly from me and have your questions answered.

Here's what you'll learn:

- The absolute most important parts of the *PT Website Secrets*™ *System* that previous students have implemented, the result of which immediately added upwards of $40K to their revenue in less than 1 year.
- The shocking reasons why your website is actually DETERRING patients from calling you.
- How one student used his website to add $2K in 2 months to his bottom line *without* spending any money on advertising.

Sign up for my next free live training if you want to see exactly how the *PT Website Secrets™ System* is being used by other physical therapy business owners like you. I want you to hear from those who came before you. I want you to see and understand that you CAN finally get new patients from your website.

At the end of the training, you'll be given a special opportunity to enroll in my signature program, *The Workshop*, where we can work together personally to transform your website, your business, and your life.

Option #2: Work With Christine in *The PTWS WORKSHOP*

The Workshop is my signature program that teaches all of the *PT Website Secrets™* Principles in-depth. It gives you everything you need to either transform your current website OR build a new one entirely from scratch. I share in significantly more detail everything you've read in this book, and what's more, I give you the practical know-how and everything you need to apply these Principles to your business. I also share with you all of my latest templates – yes, the exact one I use to build patient-generating websites for my exclusive private clientele.

The Workshop is the quickest way to get you the online website success you're looking for with the least amount of hassle. All you have to do is follow my step-by-step program – the exact one that has helped over 100 physical therapist across the world double, triple, and even increase their new patient leads tenfold! With *The Workshop* you'll stop running around begging for new referrals and finally feel like the confident business owner I know you are. You're not just another physical therapist – it's time to make that clear.

The Workshop will show you the same system Kris Winders used for *BBN Physical Therapy*'s website to add 40K to his business in one year ALONE, all from ONE BUTTON. It's the same system Paul Jones, of Jones Physical Therapy in Madisonville, LA, used to get 10 new patients via his website within 2 weeks of launching it. It's the program that self-proclaimed "tech-dinosaur", Laura McKaig, used to create and launch a brand new website, on her own, in less than 6 weeks. John Davidson applied these Principles and now gets patients calling saying, "I found your website and knew you could help me!" Cameron Dennis learned this system and in months went from having only 3-4 phone calls from his website to 3-4 calls a week! This is the new system to transform your business and your life from day one. Don't take my word for it – join The Workshop and see for yourself!"

When you join *The Workshop* you'll work with me, personally, for 8 weeks. I'll show you, step-by-step, exactly how to finally get new patients and grow your business with the internet. We'll work together to get your website where it needs to be. You'll be part of a community of physical therapists who have already gone before you, completed the program, and are eager to help newcomers achieve the same success they have.

The entire course is delivered to you via videos, worksheets, live calls with me, and the support of the amazing *PT Website Secrets*™ community! That way, you'll have everything you need to finally achieve your dreams and be the next success story.

JOIN *THE WORKSHOP* HERE:

www.ptwebsitesecretsbook.com/workshop

Here's what we'll cover together in the program:

- **You'll discover exactly how to get a successful PT website that converts visitors to new patient leads** so that you can stop worrying about where the next new patient is coming from, let alone when.
- **You'll understand exactly why** the BEST physical therapy websites give away valuable information for free AND how to implement the same strategy quickly and

easily <u>(so you don't miss out on the 85% who aren't ready to BOOK NOW)</u>!

- **You'll skip past all the mistakes and obstacles** that MOST PT practice owners make and go right to the end of the process.
- **You'll know exactly how to avoid the BIGGEST mistake** people make when writing content for their website (and why it keeps potential patients from calling your clinic)!
- **You'll have a TON more money in your pocket** when you stop losing out on all the patients you COULD be getting from your website!

If you're ready to be an action taker and get the online advantage over your competition, then this system is exactly what you've been looking for. If you don't want to waste any more time with the old ways of building websites and hustling around for referrals, then go ahead and enroll in *The Workshop* now: *www.ptwebsitesecretsbook.com/workshop*

Want to know the best part of taking *The Workshop*? I've had students have up to a 900% return on their investment... before they've even finished the program. They've told me that not only did the program change their websites and their businesses forever, but it also changed the way they think about themselves as physical therapists.

Why can't that be you? Let your website start making the difference you deserve. Contact me now for more information.

I challenge you to step outside of your comfort zone, embrace the unknown, and fight for your dream. Together, using *PT Websites Secrets*, we can do it!

Pick the option that best suits you and I look forward to seeing you in the next webinar or joining us in *The Workshop*!

To your website's success!

Christine